HALF A
HEAD

Gemma Bromley

Thanks for making me stronger ♡

Gem x

ISBN: 978-1-913479-47-3 (paperback)
ISBN: 978-1-913479-48-0 (ebook)

That Guy's House
20-22 Wenlock Road
London
England
N1 7GU
www.thatGuysHouse.com

For my son, Oscar

"I see trees of green, red roses too, I see them bloom for me and you, and I think to myself what a wonderful world"- Louis Armstrong

Acknowledgments

Firstly, I want to give a heartfelt thanks to Emma Mumford, my mentor throughout the process of writing this book, for giving me the opportunity to birth my book baby, and for seeing something in my journey that I hope will help many! An enormous glittery thanks to That Guys House publishers – the magic in making this dream become a reality, and a special mention to Jesse for keeping my work as authentic and honest as it comes. A big thanks to Sean Patrick the founder of That Guys House, I am so grateful to be part of your author family, and for this opportunity – what a privilege. To Jenifer Richards - my lovely friend, without you this book would have not made it this far, you are amazing. Thanks to my fellow authors' who ventured on this journey with me, for cheering me on – I know you will all bring out some wonderful reads. Thanks to Nye for formatting this book – so grateful, and to Solen Photography for capturing some fun filled pics of me for my website.

Thanks to one of my oldest and dearest friends Jon, for creating the most wonderful website to promote this book, for all your support and friendship over the thirty or so years. Thanks for loving me just the way I am – my fairy airy ways!

A gigantic love filled thanks to my dad, for allowing me to feature your incredibly talented pencil sketches throughout this book. They have brought my story to life and captured my words just as I see them from within. You have shaped my history, my character, to a far greater extent than you think. Dad, you are the finest, loveliest, tenderest, and most beautiful person I will ever know – and even that is an understatement.

So much thanks and love to my mum, for giving up so much of yourself to look after me, and for not once asking for time off! Thank you for remaining positive in times when the sun stopped shining for me. You never let go of my hand throughout, even when I made it harder for you to hold. You're the strongest superwomen I know, I still don't know how you did it – you're my role model.

Thanks to my sister Nicola, I could not have done this without you – I'm talking past and present, my recovery, my move to Scotland, this book – life! You told me that you will never be able to fix me, but that I would never have to face it alone, you have always been by myside. I feel so blessed to have a sister like you.

Thanks to my brother-in law Gaz, my life oracle! I am so grateful for your encouragement and support in this 18-year journey of finding myself, and showing me that life would be awfully boring being perfect, something I used to think I needed for some reason:

"they will see us waving from such great heights, come down now they'll say – but everything looks perfect from far away, come down now but we'll stay" -The Postal Service

Life is not a competition.

A big sparkly thanks to Jo and Steve, for putting your lives on hold for me (even your wedding) and being by my side throughout. Thank you for the breakdown of the medical concepts, and for keeping it real for everyone else. Thanks to my wonderful cousins Louis and Rosa, for only knowing me with a brain injury, and loving me more for it. An extra bit of glittery thanks for Jo, for writing your personal account of my accident for this book. I know you have written medical books in the past, but this one must have been the hardest! I look up to you, you have this incredible strength and passion that you exemplify in your everyday life, and I aspire to be like you.

Rainbows of gratitude for my Granny Polly – what can I say? You just get me – correction we get each other. Thank you for keeping a journal so I could write this book, and for being there for me always. To my uncle Nick – the big personality in the family, you've always encouraged me to go BIG or go home, and thanks to you, I've never gone with the latter!

So much love and thanks to all my amazing family members who have helped me through my journey of recovery, along with family friends, my friends families, work colleagues, my teachers, old school friends and strangers who prayed for me – you know who you are.

Enormity of thanks to Andy for letting me feature you in this book. If I were to write down all the reasons that I am grateful for your support throughout my accident, I'd take up far too much paper, since I'm now this eco-warrior, I'll keep it short! Everyone who knows you, knows what a great guy you are, and I am so blessed to have had you by my side at that time in my life. I was a disaster, the worst of its kind, yet you still gave me the courtesy to tell me I was beautiful – I don't think I ever said thanks until now, you're a true gentleman. A shout out to your parents and brother, who gave me a lot of support throughout – thank you.

A big thanks to Claire, what a journey we've been on, despite the tough, sometimes harrowing times the accident had on our friendship, I am glad we found each other again later in life, and that we both found closure in that moment to move on. Thank you for letting me discuss you in this book, and for being the kind person you are today.

An enormous meteorite explosion of thanks to my incredible best friend Laura – I want to thank you for being the friendship that I needed all those years ago. You changed me; you healed me, and even though I didn't know at the time, you saved me. *"You're my person"* – Greys

Enormous waves of gratitude to all the medical staff at Birmingham Sally Oak Hospital and Birmingham Queen Elizabeth Hospital, especially to Mr Whatsenburgh, for giving me a new skull and a new opportunity to live life to its fullest. More big waves of thanks to The Midlands Air Ambulance – your courageous work is making a massive difference to people's lives; it certainly did to mine.

Thanks to one amazing off-duty firefighter - Andy, you are the reason I am alive today, I will be forever grateful for what you did for me that morning. A big thanks to all the professions I have worked with over the years from Speech Therapists, Occupational Therapists, Physiotherapists, Psychiatrists, Neurologists, healthcare assistants, and anyone else who has helped me throughout the years - thank you.

Special loving thanks to my friendship seeds aka Charlotte, Helen, Rachel and Del – it is one of my highest privileges to have you lot in my world. *"The best kind of friendships are fierce lady friendships, where you aggressively believe in each other, and think the other deserves the world"* -Unknown

To my precious friend Emma, thank you for being there for me, from the first day I got to know you many moons ago at school, I knew how lucky I was because well... *"when you find people who not only tolerate your quirks but celebrate them with happy cries of ME TOO be sure to cherish them. Because those weirdos are your tribe"* – unknown

HUGE thanks to my wonderful friends I have been fortunate enough to create since moving to Scotland – you all know who you are, and if you're wondering if I am talking about you...I most certainly am.

A big colourful thanks to my special friend Rose, for letting me discuss you in this book. You are many things to me... my shrink, my motivator, my critic, my hoddit, my cheerleader, my crown fixer ...even my bin lady (laughs) BUT you are also THE best human diary that one could have - one that I can highly recommend, but unfortunately, she's not for sale! – thank you!

Thanks to my amazing friend Rich, you're one of the most interesting people I have had the privilege of meeting, and despite knowing you most of my life, you never fail to teach me something new. The one thing you always used to tell me was to be myself and to be proud – possibly the best advice from you yet!

A special thanks to my very kind friend Alysia, for befriending me when I was completely lost, both physically and emotionally (I was a not in a good place), although we see each other once in a blue moon, I know that we are each other's cheerleader's from a far!

Big thanks to Jade, for letting me talk about you in my book and discuss some terrifying school threats we both went through – thank you for being my backbone, and for sharing some difficult memories that nobody could understand but us. Lots of thanks to my friend Sam, for feeding me up, for making me laugh, for all your letters of support (I still have). Thanks to my dear friend Kelly, for being such a lovely friend in times of need. I know that you guys will be friends for life, even if we go through years without contact.

Thanks to my school friends and supporters – Natalie and Holly for being there for me in many ways, I am so grateful for that, and for all your hospital visits. Thanks to my oldest friends Heather and Emily for being there for me when I was in my recovery, when most people thought I was okay. Thanks for your kindness and support – I might have a bad memory now, but I have never forgotten that!

So much love to my beautiful friends Amber and Hannah, as you know I am very indecisive and always have trouble picking my favourite anything. BUT without a doubt, you guys are my favourite everything! I am so lucky to have met you later in my life, you bring so much love to my life.

Thanks to my amazing university professor John Irvine, you inspire me so much to go through life without your sight yet be able to see the richest colour in people – you did with me. Thank you for everything, you mean so much to me.

I want to thank Rajni and Alka for your love and support, and to your family that is full of beautiful souls. I know that Rajni would have been so proud to have read this book, he was incredibly special to me. I feel I have a second family, and I love you all so much.

Thank you to Rebekah for allowing me to feature you in this book, and for our beautiful unique friendship we have made in our crazy old world of brain injury.

Thanks to Catrina, for allowing me to discuss you in my book and to use your words, which I know will inspire many.

A HUGE thanks to the love of my life Jamie, even though we met much later in my journey, I know that we'll be taking the rest of it together – *"Real love doesn't meet you at your best. It meets you in your mess"* J.S. Park

Thank you to everyone who I have not mentioned – until now, who have supported me and loved me just the way I am.

AND…

Finally, thanks to my beautiful little boy Oscar, one day when you read this, you won't be so little, and I will be so honoured that you get to read my story! I want you to know that you are my daily inspiration, my reason for everything and my absolute joy in life:

"I carry your heart; I carry it in my heart" – E.E Cummings

Contents

Introduction

'To be nobody but yourself – in a world which is doing its best, night and day, to make you everybody else – means to fight the hardest battle which any human being can fight; never stop fighting.' – E.E Cummings

Identity

noun

1. The fact of being who or what a person or thing is.

2. The characteristics determining who or what a person or thing is.

We all know what we mean when we discuss 'identity', at least we think we do, but does it go further than the obvious? We identify someone by their name, age, career, culture, race, religion and so on. Although this is true, identity very much comes from within us. It's not our exterior make-up of how we look, what we wear, how big our house is or how flashy our car looks; it's our interior design that is handpicked by *'you'* and only you; that is the person you are in your own unique, remarkable way. It sounds straightforward when I put it like that. I have really struggled with losing and re-finding my own identity, which is, in part, why I wanted to write this book.

For over seventeen years I've been giving identity quite some thought; in fact, I've bounced the concept around my mind, back and forth, like I was Andy Murray smashing it at Wimbledon! I've learnt a lot about identity after sustaining a severe head injury and one hell of an operation that changed my life forever. I lost both my external and my internal identity in the blink of an eye: my health, my hair, my appearance, my abilities to walk, talk, eat, see, hear and remember things, my IQ, recognition of the people I loved most, and of course part of my brain. After coming out of my coma and going through seemingly endless rehabilitation, I couldn't imagine going out into the world again as this person I no longer knew.

'One of the hardest things you will ever have to do is to grieve the loss of a person who is still alive.' – Unknown

The brain is one of the most precious organs in our body. It controls everything we say, everything we do, what we think and how we feel. With it weighing less than sixteen hundred grams (that's just three pounds), the brain resembles no more than a soft, wrinkled walnut, yet despite the inauspicious appearance the human brain can store more information than all the libraries in the world, according to Richard Restak, a well-known American Clinical Professor of Neurology and author. When our brain is damaged it is referred to as 'brain injury'. 'Traumatic brain injury' (TBI) is defined by the NHS as 'a serious blow to the head or a penetrating head injury that disrupts the function of the brain'.

Not all blows to the head result in TBI, and it can vary from being 'mild', for example, a brief change in mental state or consciousness, to 'severe', for example, an extended period of unconsciousness or amnesia after injury. As if that wasn't enough for our wrinkled little walnuts to process, there is also acquired brain injury (ABI). ABI differs from TBI in its causes, but the effects of both injuries on a person's life are very similar. The National Institute of Neurological Disorders and Stroke (NINDS), explains ABI as 'an injury to the brain that is not hereditary, congenital or degenerative'. ABI can be caused by some medical conditions, including strokes, encephalitis, aneurysms, anoxia (lack of oxygen during surgery), drug overdose, near drowning, metabolic disorders, meningitis, or brain tumours.

I am thirty-five years old; half of my skull is made up from titanium plate, and I live with Traumatic Brain Injury (TBI), which has left me with a permanent disability which, although hidden, is there and always will be. I grew up in a little town called Droitwich Spa. This hidden gem of a town is in the Midlands, England, on the River Salwarpe. If any of you have ever visited Droitwich, you won't need me telling you just how special it is. It's situated on enormous deposits of salt, which is ten times stronger than seawater. Droitwich was where my journey started; it was the place that grew me, with my beautiful family and some of my oldest and dearest friends colouring the place with character. Although, naturally, people move on – like myself – the memories remain and the people in Droitwich shaped me. Every person, every experience, every memory, good or bad, has helped me to create this book. I now live in Edinburgh, and after quite some years in Scotland, I feel content in calling it my home. I moved up to escape a few demons and to find myself – isn't that what we all want to do? I knew I wouldn't find the real me staying put and always knew I would find adventure somewhere new. After completing university and after receiving a lot of job knock-backs, I managed to bag my dream job at the Royal Institute for the Blind at The Eye Pavilion in Edinburgh, and I was thrilled to start my next chapter in a new place.

I completely, one hundred percent, without a doubt manifested this job. It changed my mindset and gave me an incredible insight into the lives of partially sighted and blind people. I decided to work in sensory loss as I had such a strong intuitive calling for it; my intuition told me that I had something more to give, a way of helping others, which is all I've ever wanted to do. Who better for the job than someone who knew how it felt to lose one's identity? Whether it was sight, hearing, a limb, or the big and obvious one for me, part of the brain (though I too suffered from sight loss and I also have hearing loss in one ear), I felt well equipped to help people going through these types of losses. They all make up our identity, which for some, just like magic and without any consent, vanish overnight, leaving us to question who we are.

I find that children have an incredible, different take on identity because theirs is still under development, and nothing really matters as long as their needs are met. They don't concern themselves with their identity; often they ooze confidence naturally and aren't afraid of the world or how they appear because their own little unique identity comes only from within. It's not until our teenage years that external identity really comes into play; suddenly, we become fixated on what others think about us and how we can conform to our friendship groups: totally natural for that age. At seventeen years old, my awareness of my identity was at its peak, and having it snatched away from me was traumatic. It took me a long time to find the positives in my desperate situation. I felt depressed and I got frustrated with myself all the time – I could no longer do the things I used to be able to do in the way I wanted to. Right at the very bottom of my soul, however, buried exceptionally well, was a light, albeit a very small glow, of hope. Sometimes I was able to turn it on, and when I did, I knew it was all going to be ok.

In the beginning of my recovery, I tried very hard to appreciate the things that were going well, such as the work of the wonderful consultants who were designing and rebuilding my skull with titanium plate, and my incredibly positive and supportive family – my parents and sister, my boyfriend and my friends. Fundamentally, I was still me because I still had my personality; luckily that was something I hadn't lost – though my dad said when I was able to function normally it was like I had taken a truth drug: I was very honest about everything and perhaps over-shared, which gave us all a few giggles along the way! Coming to think of it, my friends would probably still describe me a bit like this now. I don't hold back, that's for sure! If something's not appropriately timed, you can be sure that I will let the cat out of the bag! I have grown to love this about myself, one of the many after-effects of brain injury. I like that people know I am honest and that I will always, under any circumstances, blurt out the truth, even if it leaves me cringing for days after!

When I was in hospital there wasn't much my family could turn to for help, and certainly no memoirs offering insight to families facing trauma in their lives. Later in my recovery, I was desperate to find a 'happy ever after' book from another teenager who had undergone brain surgery so that I could learn about their struggles, and how they coped with their new identity. I really needed a book that wasn't necessarily written by a celebrity or well-known author, just a bog-standard average Joe like me!

Identity comes hand in hand with confidence, which deflates quicker than ever when you look in the mirror one day liking what you see, then the next time you look you can't even bear to look at yourself because *who is that person staring back?!* In this book, I will share what I have learnt about confidence in my own life, as well as what I have learnt from growing up with a hidden disability. I want everyone to feel confident, whatever walk of life, whatever hurdles jumped or fallen. This book is about finding the courage to live the life you know you deserve; it is about empowering everyone to challenge the views of disability in today's society; it is about looking beyond external identity and reaching within to find true beauty and contentment.

'A crack does not mean you are broken; it means you were put to the test and you did not fall apart.' – Linda Poindexter

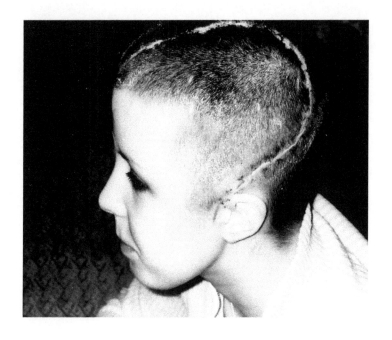

Chapter One
No Ordinary Morning

'Life is an intricate piece of tapestry; you follow a certain pattern that suddenly changes direction to create a beautiful piece of artwork. Appreciating the small yet rather large errors, that somehow fit strangely into the masterpiece.' – Stephen Bromley, 2002.

It was 26th April 2002, and I woke up to a beautiful sunny morning with the usual birds chirping. It was like any other morning – ordinary in many ways – and with a cup of tea in one hand, toast and marmite in the other, I was waiting for my friend to pick me up. Claire had just passed her driving test and to say we were excited was an understatement. I was so happy for her! We'd decided to go to McDonald's to get breakfast. After spending time in front of the mirror perfecting my hair and asking the million-dollar question of 'What top should I wear...?' (oh, the trivial things back then) I was ready to go! Little did I know this morning would be no ordinary morning; little did I know that the following two hours would change my life forever. I was about to meet my fate and boy did the Universe have a plan for me!

I remember that morning well. I had been a typical hormonal teenager and had disagreed with my mum, who didn't want me to skip maths. She had my dad on her back to talk sense into me, as he'd left for work early. Not that I was a problematic teen at all – I was no trouble for my parents. Both my sister Nicola and I were a dream when I look back now. I just really hated maths – the way it was taught made no sense to me – although I wish I'd tried harder now. Hindsight is a wonderful thing. But I wouldn't change a thing about that morning. Not one. Every moment was leading me to 'me', I just didn't know it at the time. Mum had a 'feeling', like she'd get from time to time (always right, I must admit), but I thought she was worrying for nothing and asked her to stop nagging. I selfishly walked out that morning, slamming the door behind me without saying goodbye, and I am sure leaving behind some negative energy for poor mum to soak up and carry around with her. Mum – I am sorry I did that. This book will be difficult for you to read.

I know that Mum and Dad blamed themselves for years for not putting their foot down and stopping that morning's adventure, but now they see my growth and determination, and as Dad always says, 'It's all part of the tapestry in life'. There is a lesson for everyone here though. No matter what, NEVER EVER walk out the door without a goodbye, because that old saying 'You might just get hit by a bus' could become a reality. You really could, and I really did.

I can only tell the next bit from a bird's-eye view. I prefer to believe that my life-changing experience was more than a sudden black hole of nothing. I believe part of me somehow rose from within and I became my own guardian angel. Perhaps it was everything I learnt in the aftermath and the scary facts I had to face from my doctors. I guess I will never know, but what I am sure of is this: when you are in a critical condition your body shuts down because the pain is too much to experience, but you are still in there: you are fighting like a trooper, you're in flight mode and every second counts. To those of you reading this book that have or are going through something similar, I hope this book gives you courage and strength to restart life again after trauma. I hope it helps you to believe in life's magic when all hope fades away from you.

At the neurological level, a coma is like a deep sleep. Clinically speaking, the brain is dormant, in a persistent sleep-like state. Someone in a coma is unresponsive to light, sound and verbal communication, and incapable of initiating purposeful action. Every brain injury is different, but generally, brain injury is classified according to the Glasgow Coma Scale (GSC), which is a neurological scale that aims to give a reliable and objective way of recording someone's state of consciousness. Severe head injury is classed as a GCS of 8 or less; moderate head injury is a GCS of 9-12; and mild head injury is GCS of 13-15. I had a GCS of 3 when the Air Ambulance reached me. I was in a bad way, treading the fine line between slipping into death or staying.

Claire and I were coming back from our McDonald's trip, heading back to Droitwich Spa Sixth Form where we were studying for our A-levels. Suddenly, our car jerked a few times. I remember that well and laughed it off, as these things happen, especially to new drivers. As we approached the T-junction joining a busy 60 mph (now a

40 mph) speed limit road in Fernhill Heath, a cosy village near our hometown, a bus was coming up the road and flashed its lights at us. Claire pulled out and as she did, the bus hit us, spinning our car across the road as the impact pushed our car in the opposite direction.

On impact I had come out of the top part of my safety belt, subsequently hitting my head on every window of the car. A lady driving behind us witnessed this and told the medics I looked like a rag doll getting thrown around the car, hitting my head over and over. An off-duty fire officer, who I later found out was called Andy (the same name as my boyfriend at the time), was having brunch in a nearby pub next to the road and heard the impact from inside. He came out to investigate. He could see Claire was in shock, not making much sense, with what appeared to be broken collar bone from my head smashing onto her body, and blood, lots and lots of blood. It must have been so scary for Claire to see it all with her own eyes; I'm sure she has a very different account of what happened, and I am grateful that she supports me now to tell my story.

I was lying in Claire's lap, bleeding from my mouth, ears and nose, my breathing was shallow and gurgling, and Andy said he knew he had to move me to clear my airways. He cut me free from the bottom half of my safety belt and sat me upright because he knew an ambulance just wouldn't make it in time to save me. To this day, I am so grateful for Andy's quick, professional thinking.

Andy wrote in the accident report: 'I didn't see the accident; I heard the collision from upstairs in the Bull Inn

Pub. Initially, I thought it was a minor accident because the noise of the impact was not that loud. I decided to go and see if everyone was ok, but I found the two girls in the car had been injured. I could see the driver had blood on her face and was obviously distressed. I then went around the other side as I could see the passenger lay in the driver's lap bleeding quite heavily. My initial thoughts were not to move her because of possible spinal injury, but after going into the car and listening to her breathing she was obviously struggling and she was making a gurgling, choking noise. I decided to lift her to the upright position and clear her airway.'

If he hadn't have been close by that day, I wouldn't be here writing my story, which is why Andy, if you're reading this, thank you, you're one of Earth's Angels and we're lucky to have you.

It was late morning and Mum was at work. Even now, all these years later, she says she had a feeling something bad had happened. It was around eleven in the morning when the police arrived at her work; working at the Crown Prosecution Service, Mum was used to speaking to the police, so she didn't think anything of it. However, when they asked if she was my mum, she knew it was bad news. One police officer told her I had been in a road traffic accident involving a bus and had hit my head, that she needed to come to hospital with them immediately. Mum said her legs gave way as she fell forwards and remembers saying *'Not her head'*. The rest for Mum and my family was a blur. My sister Nicola was studying psychology at Bristol University and hadn't yet been told. My absolute rock and incredible long-term boyfriend at the time, Andy, gave up everything to come and support us. Mum called Dad, who was at work at the time, and he came straight away. Dad's work colleague kindly drove to Bristol to fetch my sister. The way people pull together through tragic events really warms me. I had people I didn't know reaching out, praying for me; I even had some holy water sent across from India. My parents didn't want Nicola to panic and didn't give her all the facts, but she knew it was serious if she had to leave university to come to the hospital, along with having an escort fetch her that she did not know. My sister's boyfriend, Gaz, who I'm now lucky enough to call my brother-in-law, also dropped his studying at Stafford University so he could be by my side and support us all. The doctors had told my parents that they needed to prepare themselves and contact all the family to come to the hospital as soon as possible to give them the chance to say goodbye.

'You got wires, goin' in, you've got wires, comin' out of your skin, you got tears making tracks, I got tears, that are scared of the facts.' – Athlete; 'Wires'

My parents said they couldn't take any photos of me at the time, as if I had died that day; they didn't want to remember me that way. I have some photos that were taken of me later in my recovery, which I have shared in this book. My family said I had swelled so much I was unrecognisable; my weight went from eight stone to fourteen stone because the swelling was so bad. My sister described me as *'wires'*: all she could see were wires going in and out of my body, and all she could make out was the tip of my nose. Nicola arrived at hospital and navigated herself to the intensive care ward. She wasn't prepared for what she saw, and she always says the chart hit song at that time 'Wires' by Athlete described exactly what it felt like for her that day, and sure enough, running down corridors, through automatic doors was quite the reality for her.

We all know that saying – that Grandmas are like Grand-Angels – and thank goodness for mine. I owe big thanks to my amazing Granny Polly for keeping a journal of my accident. She recorded my progress which has been invaluable to me in writing this book, but she was also my rock and still is. Good old Granny Polly, she's my best friend – now how many people can say that about their Granny? She didn't leave my side. I'll talk more about family later BUT she deserves a special mention.

I was hooked up on a life support machine in intensive care which, along with a blood transfusion, was keeping me alive. The doctors needed to relieve the pressure building on my brain from the swelling. They inserted a vent into my forehead, but this failed to work. Twenty-four hours later my parents signed a document of consent for an emergency craniotomy. In non-medical terms, this meant that I needed to have my left bone flap removed. This was to allow my brain to swell and relieve the pressure held inside my skull. That same day, I had a CT scan which indicated there was 'an intensive acute left subdural haematoma with some foci of haemorrhage in the underlying cerebral cortex' – which, in short, means that I had a blood clot on my brain and a bleed. My medical report went on to say that the contusions, meaning bruises, were also noted in the left cerebral hemisphere and tissue swelling over the right temporo-parietal region – this was referring to the different areas of my brain that had been affected.

A subsequent CT scan stated that the blood from the subdural haematoma had tracked to the back of my skull, which wasn't good news. Whilst in theatre, my neurosurgeon was able to see that there were alterations in the structure of my brain and superficial contusions (bruises) over the Wernicke's area. For those of you who aren't aware, the Wernicke's area is the region of the brain that is important for language development; it helps us with understanding speech and using the correct words to express our thoughts. The Broca's area was also altered – this is the motor speech area of the brain and it helps in movements required to produce speech. Interestingly, the Broca's area is named after Paul Broca, who discovered this region whilst treating a patient, who was referred to as 'Tan'. Tan could understand spoken language but was unable to produce any coherent words and could only say 'Tan'. After his death, Broca conducted a post-mortem on Tan's brain and found that he had lesions (abnormal tissue) in the left frontal lobe, which led him to conclude that this area of the brain was responsible for speech production. People with damage to this area experience Broca's aphasia which is a challenge I face daily; I will be discussing this later in my book.

Giving the go-ahead for the operation was the biggest decision my parents have ever had to make. The chance of the operation being a success, and that I would survive, was 50/50. The huge risk was that I might not regain normal neurological levels. In the dark hole my family felt they had entered, they believed I had got this far and told the medical team to do whatever they had to do to save my life. Mum said she read through the small print of all the complications that could happen and was terrified. Dad said he felt like he was in space, everything happening in slow motion, rotating up in the air. Luckily for me, my family's positive attitude and optimistic outlook lit the skies above and kept me fighting inside my unconsciousness. I am sure that having family and close friends who so quickly adapted their own thoughts into positives was half the road to my recovery. After all, nothing mirrors your quality of life more than the power of one's own thoughts, and how that can be transferred to others around you can make all the difference.

Following surgery, the consultant neurosurgeon told my family that it was the largest part of bone flap he had removed in someone of my age. My family recalls the operation to be the longest day of their lives. After ten hours, they learnt that it had been a success, but for the next seven days, I remained in a coma. The doctors couldn't predict how I would be if I woke up. For my family and friends, it was a waiting game and the whole world stopped around them. My sister described it like waiting for a cocoon to unravel; they were waiting for me to wake up and spread my wings so together we could rebuild our lives.

In order to tell my story with as much accuracy as possible, I wanted to highlight the same story from a family member's perspective. I asked my aunty, Dr Jo Bromley, to discuss and relive her own account of this day, as just like everything in life, no one person will share the same account, which makes for an interesting notation.

'*Looking at you now you would never know.*' – Athlete;
'Wires'

I was at work when I got the call. My mum rang to say I had better come back to Birmingham as Gemma had been in a car accident. She knew that Gemma had been airlifted to hospital and that she needed to be cut out of the car. 'There's not a scratch on her, apparently,' she said, and I knew this meant she had sustained a head injury and that life as she knew it would never be the same.

There are lots of memories I have from that day, like stills from a film. I remember walking into the hospital and seeing my brother (Steve), and sister-in-law (Pam) looking lost, struggling to process what was happening. We were sat in a waiting room next to intensive care and it was explained that the first twenty-four hours would be crucial. Then the next twenty-four after that. If Gemma survived seventy-two hours post-accident, she was much more likely to live. When I first saw her, she looked exactly as if she was asleep, but had swelled so much she wasn't recognisable. She still had dried blood and dirt in her hair: staff explained they wanted to touch and stimulate her as little as possible so that her brain had very little to process. But it quickly became clear that the pressures in her head were increasing at a rapid rate.

In no time her parents were faced with a terrible decision, and had to consent to let the surgeons remove half her skull and some of her brain that had separated onto the skull to give the rest room to swell up and hopefully start to heal. Without the operation, she would have died. With it, she still might still have died but there was a chance of healing, and really it was the only option to take. Neurosurgeons of varying rank came to talk through the operation and risks. Fortunately, my partner is a doctor, and he translated into words we could understand what was going to happen, repeating again and again what they had said so we could process it better. Just before the operation, my brother Nick's partner, who was a hairdresser, cut Gemma's hair for the last time in preparation. It was these kindnesses and care that helped everyone.

Time stood still during those seventy-two hours as the enormity of Gemma's injuries started to become apparent. We did draw strength from each other and from another set of startled, grieving relatives who were there to support their husband and father. Two of us were allowed by Gemma's bed in critical care at any one time and we took shifts, swapping in and out when Pam and Steve needed to eat or rest. Finally, I think after about a week, they lifted the induced coma and we held our breaths.

I am a clinical psychologist and know that the one thing you can never predict is how someone will recover after a head injury. The smallest insult to the brain, the shortest concussion, can leave someone with significant difficulties. I remembered the famous case of Phineas Gage, who we were taught about as undergraduates. He managed to get a railway sleeper stuck through his head but carried on, undaunted, with his life. The point is, you can never tell until someone wakes up and starts their recovery, and even then, you can never be sure what they will relearn.

I knew that the amount of frontal lobe damage Gemma had incurred would be crucial. The frontal lobe is where your personality sits, your ability to moderate and reason. Frontal lobe injury can lead to painful changes in personality, make you more sexualised or impulsive. There were hundreds of questions but nothing anyone could answer. We just didn't know; we sat, and we waited, cocooned in our individual numbness.

I think, with hindsight, the professional knowledge I had made me doubt how much Gemma could recover, although I remained hopeful. But her mum and dad were resolute that they would take a day at a time and stay positive and as it turned out, they were absolutely right.

When she first opened her eyes, her gaze was unfocused and unfixed. She only seemed to be able to move one side of her body and did so repeatedly and unceasingly. The nurses created a tent of sheets over her bed with pegs so she could continually move her one arm and leg, as she seemed driven to do. She was unable to swallow water, as she would have choked, and was fed intravenously. I remember learning that the brain uses the most calories of any organ in the body so when it was trying to repair itself, she needed a super calorific diet. Despite this, she quickly lost weight.

Every day, we watched and waited and talked to her. We hugged each other and tried to make sense of it. I think we all carried a weight within us that would not lift. Gemma's sister, Nicola, had been suddenly removed from her university study, not knowing when she'd be back, if at all that year. Gemma's boyfriend was too young and naive really to grasp that she was not going to get better next week or next month or next year. This was clearly going to be a long journey.

It is difficult to relive this part of our family experience, partly because it is hard to go over such an awful time but partly because the Gemma from those days is not the Gemma that is writing this book. She has changed over the years, matured, and she lives such a full life that it is almost inconceivable to look back through the years at her seventeen-year-old self and think that we did not know if she would speak again, or walk again, or what her level of independence would be.

Support for Readers

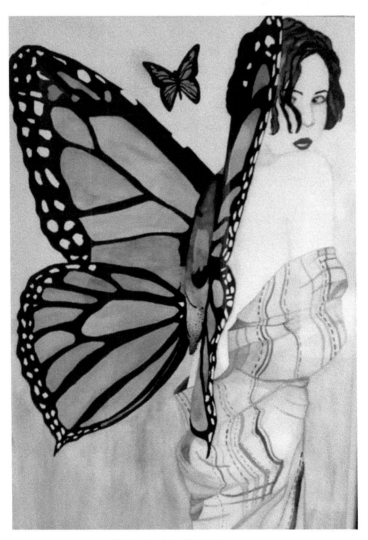

Illustrated by Nicola Deacon

If my family could offer one bit of advice, it wc
to stay connected to each other. This is the best way ᵕ.
supporting each other. Exhaustion is a common aspect
of experiencing family trauma. As a family, we worry
about the scary facts that we just can't control when a
loved one is fighting for their life in intensive care. We
can start to fall into the ugly black hole of worrying,
worries that we needn't have. We have absolutely no
control over what the future holds; creating negative
possibilities from our worries can mentally drain us.
Worries will start to bounce off the small confined
waiting room walls, the place where you all sit watching
the clock ticking, waiting and pacing. Here are some tips
for finding your waiting room zen, things that certainly
helped my family:

Mindfully prepare for the waiting period

Make sure you are hydrated with lots of fluids and warm
drinks with sugar to keep energy levels high. Take it in
turns to go to the hospital canteen; you might not feel
like eating, but if you become poorly, you will be no help
for your loved one, and they need you to stay healthy
so you can stay strong for them. Support each other by
taking it in turns to eat together. Bring in foods that will
keep energy levels healthy – things like oat bars if you
are unable to eat much.

Be friendly and smile

You might not feel like smiling, but remembering to
be pleasant to the medical staff at the hospital not

only brings you back to the present moment but also creates a better support network for your family and your loved one. This may seem a no-brainer, but some people (understandably) turn on their unfriendly autopilot mode when they are dealing with upsetting and uncomfortable situations.

Show compassion

By expressing compassion towards other family members waiting in the room with you, you will create a warmer environment. This is important; it's a sensitive time for everyone and it will help strengthen your support network further, especially if you share a waiting room with other families you do not know. You never know, you may just adopt a whole new family by doing this; my family certainly did. Remember they too are feeling the same emotions as you, and your support will be appreciated.

Carefully consider social media engagement

Social media is all around us these days, although not so much back in the days during my hospital stay, which I am positively grateful for. However, nowadays we can't escape social media, so for those of you who find it useful to update people on Facebook, may I warn you that it can simultaneously become very stressful. Now, listen up, because the important thing here is this: IT'S OK NOT TO HAVE THE ENERGY TO RETURN MESSAGES AND CALLS. THIS IS LIFE AND DEATH. PEOPLE WILL HAVE TO WAIT.

When we face trauma, we tend to close off and disappear into a mist of hopelessness. But there are ways to help get through the hard times. Nominating key roles and drawing on your external support network can make all the difference, and everyone will want to help. Below is a list of roles you could apply to people within your support network.

I. **The Social Communicator**

This person is someone you trust, who can cope with returning all the calls the family receives and who will message and update people as and when they need to. This person may, for example, reach out to your employer, school, friends, neighbours and so on.

II. **The Feeder**

Identify someone in the family that will make sure everyone eats and drinks. In our case, as mentioned above, we met an incredible family in the waiting room who became our extended support and second family, and luckily for us, they were feeders! This brings me back to my point that in showing compassion to others in the waiting room, we can open doors to even more support for each other that may be everlasting.

III. **The Helper**

This could be a neighbour you trust or a close friend — someone that understands the demands of the trauma you are all experiencing, who can help with keeping your home running if, like my parents, you are in the hospital 24/7. For example, help with things such as feeding your pet, walking the dog/s, staying on top of the laundry, washing dishes that may still be lying in your sink, and helping with cooking so that when you do get home for short periods you have food ready to go, especially if you are facing weeks or even months of hospital time. This person may run the duster around your home or keep on top of post. A disorganised home environment makes an already stressful situation seem more chaotic, but a clean home with all errands ticked off will help you create space in your mind.

IV. **The Mindful One**

We forget when we face trauma that we have to take care of ourselves too. With everything going on, we need that one person who can keep us calm, distract us from thinking the worst and keep spirits high. This person will also persuade you to get sleep and exercise and ensure your overall general self-care is still strong. It's no surprise that we don't want to move from the waiting room in case we miss something. We worry that the worst will happen if we leave. Having that one person that allows you to feel content in the knowledge that 'it'll be ok' to go home and shower, or pop to the cafe, is crucial.

My family were able to share these jobs, but this isn't the case for everyone. If you don't have a supportive network around you, here are a few tips on how to manage without.

1. Hospital staff will be able to support you, along with the reablement support team.

2. Charities such as the Salvation Army may be able to help. I recently read an article about the acts of kindness that workers at the Salvation Army do for

others. One of the workers commented that people often see the Salvation Army as their 'next of kin', especially the elderly, but it is a charity open to help all, and certainly worth contacting if you feel alone.

3. Ask the nursing team about the befriending scheme that hospitals have in place, run by volunteers. Having someone to talk to for the family member and the patient being cared for creates a much better outlook, and means you can count on support from others, so please do not be afraid to ask. Visits for your loved one in hospital so you can get some respite will give them something to look forward to, will help them with their recovery progress, and will keep them company. I would recommend doing a mind board with a volunteer, to help you feel on top of things at home so you can prioritise looking after your loved one in hospital, because without help you will suffer.

Salvation Army contacts

UK & Republic of Ireland Office: (020)73674500

Worldwide: https://www.salvationarmy.org/ihq/zones

And finally, as you read further into this book, you'll notice that I love to quote. So, I shall end this chapter with a powerful one:

'Make up your mind that no matter what comes your way, no matter how difficult, no matter how unfair, you will do more than simply survive. You will thrive.'
– Joel Osteen

Chapter Two
Angel in a Coma

'Gemma sustained a very serious head injury, as you may notice on the scan, she has a great defect.' – Mr Jatavallabhula, 25.07.2002

Nobody knows what it's like to be in a coma: do we plunge into a deep sleep of infinity? Or are we dormant, unaware of the outside space around us? For me, being in a coma was like being in a safe bubble, looking out in a blurry dream of my unconsciousness. Next to me in the intensive care unit lay my dear friend Rajni, fighting for his life; we were strangers in the empirical world, but we became family in the unconscious realm. Rajni woke up before me but he was adamant that whilst he was in his coma, he recalls seeing my face come to him in his unconscious sleep. He said I told him to eat, and that I would peel him fruit and feed him, he said he could taste the fruit, feel the texture and that his dry mouth was watered by the juice. Rajni said he could hear my voice telling him to eat to keep his strength up, and to keep fighting the infection that was busy poisoning his organs. Rajni was Hindu and he strongly believed I was his angel, that I visited him to help him stay alive when he was close to giving up. I say this in past tense, as

29

he sadly lost his battle to cancer last year, which broke our hearts into tiny pieces. As mentioned earlier on in Chapter One, Rajni and his family became marvellous friends with my family, and as noted in the support section of the chapter, his family were our 'feeders', our extended family, and our support network, and they helped my family cope with the long wait whilst Rajni and I were both treading that fine line. Alka, Rajni's wife, noticed my parents weren't eating or sleeping and took on their worry as if it was her own. Alka started to make meals for my family and took them into hospital to make sure they kept their strength up. She'd make delicious homemade Indian snacks. Obviously, sharing food with others is one of the most common forms of giving in Hinduism, referred to as *anna dana*. My family and I will always have respect and gratitude for Rajni's family. They are so caring and sincere, and even over a decade later, they still bring us an experience of peace and laughter. Without their support, our spirits wouldn't have stayed as high as they did.

I always say that life is magic; well, it must be in order to explain the incredible people I have so gratefully acquired in the years post-accident. I am obviously a firm believer in fate – I mean, how could I not be?! I always say that people come into your path for a reason, a season or for a lifetime. Certainly, my accident has opened me up to a zen of spiritual belief, a positive outlook on literally everything, and that even the ugliest situations can be transformed into, as Dad says, 'a beautiful masterpiece', and I have learnt that by finding my zen, my inner peace got me to the 'half a head' 99.9% fully recovered person I am today, minus my brain injury of course. But, let's not beat around the bush here, it took a long time, a very long time to recover. Now, where was I? Oh yes ...

I remember seeing an elephant in my unconsciousness. I saw it a lot in my hospital stay; it would walk up to me and stare then turn and walk away. It was bright blue, and it was enormous. You could argue that as I was on a lot of morphine, and spaced out much of the time, I was completely tripping ... but was I? It's bizarre how Rajni recalls seeing my face whilst he was in his coma, and I see an elephant, one of the Gods in Hinduism, 'Ganesha' the elephant-headed god of protection. I learnt later in my recovery that my boyfriend's parents had bought me a blue elephant, the exact colour of the one I saw while in my coma. How would I know, how could I have known?

It still didn't add up or make any sense to me, so I researched other people's experiences and found from Mindell, 2004 that individual reports of those in a coma, who are nearing death, have a rich inner life where they are open to opportunities for deep inner experiences. These include exploring the meaning of life, finishing off old business, and making spiritual connections. There is a report which states that there is a common misconception that once a patient is in a coma, unresponsive and very close to death, nothing is happening. The report points out that we attend to that individual's personal cares and then leave that person to fight for themselves. Interestingly, new research reveals that those in a coma do register what is going on around them but are unable to respond in the usual manner. I read that when connecting with someone in a deep coma, even the tiniest of signs can be doorways into the other's experience. Signs such as twitching, swallowing, eye movement, changes in heart rate, breathing, flickers, muscle tension and skin changes. In some cases, these signs have been helpful as a simple way to communicate. Let's face it, being in a coma can be lonely. For me, I had my family next to me 24/7, which I am sure kept me fighting inside. My mum would bathe my fingertips with the holy water that had kindly been sent to me from India. However, my family were told to do very little touching, as my brain didn't want to be overstimulated, but when they could, they'd gently hold my hand and talk to me. I read later in my recovery something that really stuck in my head. It was from a leaflet I found in the hospital whilst in a waiting room, written by a hospice. It stated that hospice workers nearly always report that people in a coma need and appreciate body contact, especially if they have been in hospital for a long period of time.

Eight days after I woke from my coma, I opened my eyes. I hadn't moved any part of my body and was in a sedated state. My family and Andy were naturally all feeling very fragile and emotional at the time. They didn't know if I would fully return as the Gemma they once knew, and to make it even more difficult to contend with, neither did the doctors. Mum had started to make plans in her confused, devastated mind to leave her job and care for me 24/7 and was adamant I would not be put into care. The doctors stuck to the facts. They did not dress up the outcome with rainbows and butterflies of how my future would look; they told my family I may not ever come back and were very straight from day one. My uncle Steve, a doctor himself, was able to take the medical meanings and translate them to my family in a way that didn't sound so scary. They were so lucky to have him. My aunty Jo (who is more of a big sister than aunty), also a doctor, was able to help with the medical jargon and scary facts when Steve was not around, but it was much more close to the bone for Jo, and her mind wasn't really in the right place, as she too was scared of the facts.

At that time, I must have represented some sort of zombified state to my family; I would appear to be 'staring into nothing' my sister recalls, but I remember seeing people sitting around my bed. I can't remember noticing anyone in particular at that time, but Gran noted in her journal that I seemed to be eye-scanning for what she thought was Andy. Gran has always had an innate ability to be very intuitive when it came to me, so I am sure she would have been spot on. My point is that, despite the doctor's opinion, it was unlikely I would be the person they once knew; I was still very much inside that zombified appearance of mine. Andy was my first 'proper' love; it was young love moulded together into a beautiful friendship, and my family adored him – and still do – after sticking by us. I am delighted to have been in touch with Andy recently through some social media stalking! Despite him not using these platforms, his friends came to the rescue! I wanted to ask for his permission to talk about the time in space we shared together, with it being such a challenging time. Having not really been in touch with him for many years, I was delighted to learn the warming news of his first baby, and of course, he was extremely supportive of me telling my story to help others in similar situations.

Voiceless and quadriplegic for days, I knew I had to get in the mindset of achieving small goals to show everyone that I was going to be ok. Nine days on from my craniotomy, the day after waking up from my coma, I was able to breathe for myself and was taken off ventilation. I started to make very tiny movements in my left arm. Although this was good news for everyone, I progressed from a vegetated state into a different state of impaired consciousness. My head and body were very swollen, and I still didn't look like me. I had completely lost my identity, but I didn't notice this until I was much further into my recovery. Gran noted some days later that I pulled my monitor leads out with my left hand. I remember doing something like this – I hated having so many wires going in and out of my skin, I felt claustrophobic, and they were painful. The doctors and my family were over the moon that I had the strength to do this. I was making contact, I was making a show for everyone saying, 'Guys, you know what ... here I am.' I was still paralysed on my right side, but that didn't stop me. For the doctors and my family, my movement was irrational; it was like my brain was telling my body to move but it was trapped and couldn't make sense of what to do, therefore it reacted randomly with no proper function. Sadly, these movements didn't show my brain was functioning normally and this, for everyone, was terrifying. If you know me, you'll know I am quite the determined little mite: I don't give up on the first, second or even third hurdle. Like I mentioned earlier, I was 'in there' and I was desperate to make contact – I just couldn't.

Have you ever dreamt you are trying to run somewhere to get away from something chasing you? But you can't put one foot in front of the other – you're effectively glued to the spot even though your unconscious mind state is shouting 'RUN' ... Well, that is the only way I can describe how it felt for me.

I remember being desperate for water. I wanted it so much I had recurring dreams about water most nights, which satisfied my thirst for a short time, but it wasn't enough. Eight days or so later, I spotted my sister holding a bottle of water and as she leant down to give me a kiss, I grabbed hold of her long brown hair and tried (albeit not very well) to pull myself up. I wasn't aware she was my sister; I just saw the water in her hand and boy did I want that drink. Everyone was astonished, they couldn't believe their eyes. Having shown very little movement up to that point and then suddenly summoning the energy to grab her hair with one hand was cause for a huge celebration. I showed to everyone that I was aware of what water was and its purpose. I remember being given thickened water instead, which I remember to this day. Its consistency was revolting. For any of you who have had the unfortunate opportunity to drink this – you never forget It, do you? It tasted like the paste they use at the dentist when they take impressions of your teeth ... you know, the one that ends up all over your face, which of course you don't realise until you get home and look in the mirror! I needed to have thickened water to reduce the risk of choking, medically referred to as dysphagia, which is basically when you're at an increased risk of aspiration pneumonia because the fluid consumed may inadvertently enter your lungs. However, the distant dream of drinking water was the least of my difficulties that I needed to conquer, and I remained on thickened water for the next few months.

On the 4th of May, I managed to conquer slight movement in my right leg, but nothing in my arm. It is very common for people who have sustained a head injury to lose the use of their right side. On impact of the accident, I damaged all areas of my brain, so my symptoms of having an acquired brain injury were not as straightforward as might have been the case for others. The brain has two hemispheres, the left and right hemispheres. The left hemisphere controls things like language and speech, and as discussed in Chapter One, this is where the Wernicke's area sits. The right hemisphere controls your cognitive functioning. Damage to the right side results in impaired memory, attention deficit, altered creativity and music perception, along with poor reasoning.

As we have discovered, brain injury differs from person to person; each injury comes with its own assortment of impediments to manage, but prevailing them one at a time has unfailingly led me to discover how determined I was to find the person I knew I was. To make it all more bleak, an injury to the right side of the brain results in decreased control over left-sided body movements. This is known as 'left neglect', meaning inattention to the left side of the body. I struggled with this in my recovery. I had no spatial awareness, so much that you could see me veering to the right side; my family used to prop me up straight but then it wasn't too soon before I flopped over again. I would be in a physio session and topple over to my right, because I wasn't aware of the left side of my body. It was horrendous; I would walk into things that were on my left and not even realise they were there.

Even now, all these years later, my partner is forever asking me where I get all my bruises from! I still have difficulty with my spatial awareness, albeit on a smaller scale. Dr Paresh Malhotra, a senior lecturer in neurology at Imperial College London sums it up so well in his research; he said, 'I cannot describe how the world looks to neglect patients; part of the reason it's so difficult is because we don't really appreciate how the world looks ourselves. We think it's just a nice screen and you can see everything, but that's something your brain is computing and telling you you're seeing. In fact, you're attending to specific things at specific times. Your eyes are darting all over the place, but you have a sensation of a static world.'

Later, in May, I managed the slightest movement in my right arm. My dad started to play music I had liked before the accident. He would get me to listen to it through some soft headphones, and Gran noted I seemed aware of this and appeared to be trying to help my dad get the headphones in, though they couldn't be sure with my irrational movements. Gran seemed positive in her journal; this day seemed to be a good day for me. An entry dated 8th May indicated that I was restless and pulled out my catheter – ouch, I went on to do this more times than I can count! I was not orientated in time, place, or person and couldn't verbalise words. By the following week, I was moved to the trauma ward, after I had satisfied my incredible doctor that I was able to squeeze his hand in response to some questions. Gran noted that I knew when I was uncomfortable or when I had soiled myself, which was a remarkable milestone in comparison to what I had been like.

Jo put together a memory book for me with specific photos of people in my life at that time – photos of my parents, my family, my sister and Gaz, along with my school friends. Gran noted that I touched Jo's nose and wiped my eyes with one hand; she was sure I had shown empathy, and that told them that my brain was functioning as it should, giving the correct emotions at the right time. I still hadn't pinpointed anyone who had visited me in my family, but it was noted that I tried to wave goodbye to Andy, so perhaps I recognised him. It was too soon to tell.

My family said I would get myself all tangled up in my wires because I was still moving irrationally with no order of control. The doctors were still unsure how much brain damage I would have and whether I would be paralysed. As always, my parents chose not to believe that being paralysed was going to be an option – they remained extremely positive, and Gran reported that they'd always smile around me, even though I couldn't smile back, or appear to even notice. She wrote that Mum would discuss the normalities of life with me, she would comment on the weather outside, what was going on in the news, or make a joke about something that had happened to her that day; even though I didn't smile or really make any connection back, I am sure that her one-way conversations with me made me smile from within.

The big day was on 9th May, which Gran called the miracle day in her journal! This day still and always will make my dad an emotional wreck – and frankly, who can blame him? My right hand was stronger by this time, and as Dad leant forward to insert the headphone in my ear, I whispered 'Dad' in the faint voice I had back then, and then gave him a kiss, or as Gran described, a bite, but I am certain it was supposed to be a kiss! Dad said it was the best day of his life. He ran out of the room and announced to the nurses proudly and in tears 'She said my name … she said my name,' and everyone was delighted and clapped. It was an enormous relief that I was there in mind and body, that I was fully there and didn't have long-term amnesia. Dad said it was like when I was first born: the pure joy he felt back then all came flooding back to him. I have always been a Daddy's Girl; don't get me wrong, I am very close to my mum with an unbreakable bond, BUT my dad is one of a kind. We're rooted deeply and back then he knew me better than I knew myself! Dad's a bit of a clown; he always manages to make me laugh, even when I'm at my lowest, and this was especially apparent throughout my recovery. I am sure you've all heard the quote 'Behind every great laughter is a truly incredible Dad' – I rest my case! That same day, I recognised Andy, and kissed Gran on her nose! This day was a good day; I had jumped over my first obstacle, recovery was looking good, and spirits were flying higher than you could possibly imagine!

Support for Readers

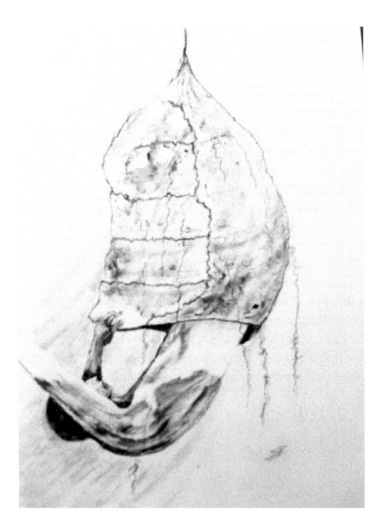

Illustrated by Steve Bromley

Communicating with someone in a coma

Below, I have simplified some ideas from Kay Ryan, 2010, along with some helpful tips my family practised with me. For those of you who don't know, Kay Ryan is a well-established author and psychotherapist and has a long-term interest in how dreams and dream-like experiences assist us through life's transitions. She is the spiritual support co-ordinator at her local hospice. Her book *Doorways into Dying: Innovative Teaching for End of Life* presents techniques and tools for communicating with those in out-of-ordinary states of consciousness, such as dementia, coma, or dying.

Be present.

Talk to them constantly; tell them you are going to touch, for example, their finger, their wrist, their arm, and so on.

Pace the rhythm of their breathing, pressing down gently each time they breathe in. You could say something like 'I can feel your breath, I am here right next to you and I am breathing with you.'

Notice your own reactions and feelings. You might feel over-emotional and that's ok; tell them how you feel, but remember to end the conversation with a positive message.

Watch for feedback, for small signs and changes to the body. If you get a sign like an eye movement, try to communicate by this, it might not work but try to work with it – what have you got to lose?

41

When connecting to the patient and they exhale, speak softly in rhythm of their breathing, near their ear. You might want to say something like 'Hello, it's me, I am here with you today and I love you. In a minute I am going to touch your arm,' then relax your touch when they exhale, like the suggestion earlier but adding more description.

In order to make the patient know they're not alone, you must keep conveying what you are doing, for example, a statement such as 'I am following the rate of your breathing; I want to follow everything that happens to you, this will help me to find a way to communicate with you better,' or you could describe other patients in beds nearby and convey positive descriptions. So, for example, you could say 'Next to you is a lady, who is doing so well; she's just like you but she's not giving up' – staying positive is key. By doing the above we can only hope that it will encourage the person to become more aware of themself.

Have normal conversations about anything you want to say – tell a joke, read the news, whatever you do is fine; they just need to know you're there. You might not get a response through signs, for example, there might not be any changes in the breathing rhythm when you talk, but that's ok – keep talking, it will help.

Play their favourite music through some soft headphones. Insert one headphone into an ear and have the sound set to low.

Play podcasts, the news, the weather and any other daily announcements.

Sing to them, and say something like 'Can you remember that song? We used to sing it all the time together'.

Read to the patient. This could be a book, a newspaper, a trashy magazine or even a television guide. Discuss programs they used to like to watch, for example, keep them updated on their beloved Coronation Street!

'Never give up on someone you love, life can go from zero to one hundred – it just requires a bit of time.'
– Unknown

Memory book

This can be a useful tool to help someone who has lost part or all of their memory; this is especially helpful for brain injury survivors. It can contain photos of people, people's names, photos of places, favourite hobbies and so on. It's important to keep it relatively plain, with little writing: too much detail can cause overload for the person.

https://www.dementia.co.uk/products/how-to-make-a-memory-book

Chapter Three
Grey Matter

'Mind is not in any one place. Every cell in this body has its own intelligence. The brain is sitting in your head, but the mind is all over the place.'
- Sadhguru

Brain injury has been called the 'silent epidemic' because public recognition of it is extremely low despite the staggering number of people who are injured each year. In the UK alone there are an estimated 350,000 people admitted to hospital with various brain injuries, from road traffic accidents (like with my own experience), to assaults, day-to-day accidents such as falling down the stairs, falling off a ladder, and work-related accidents. Then there are vascular disorders such as stokes, one of the biggest causes of brain injury. The number of brain injuries is on the rise.

People often do recover physically from their injuries. However, survivors and their families have to face adjusting psychologically to a lasting impairment as a result of brain injury. Often this includes cognitive and communicative difficulties, but the social and emotional factors can present a greater burden, with reports of a greater rate of depression among survivors. This is not only difficult to experience for everyone involved but can also slow down the person's overall recovery, which is why I did my best to stay positive.

Now, let's not get all gloomy here; not all of those with brain injuries experience a negative outlook on life, and contrary to what some professionals might expect, brain injury can actually be a source of positive personal growth. This has certainly been the case for me. My brain injury has improved my philosophy on life and helped me to make stronger personal relationships with others, not to mention that it has enhanced my quality of life. I am so much more appreciative of things now, little acts of kindness, the very small details in everything I can always see and be grateful for, and this is a liberating position to be in. So, why do some brain injury survivors recover with a better frame of mind, whilst others find it harder? Now, don't get me wrong – I have been to hell and back in my recovery, but the key for me was to take each day and do my very best. Instead of fixating on 'what's wrong', I built my internal strength – building on 'what's strong'. It's a no-brainer, really, but flipping the scenario around to make it how you want it to be is half your battle to recovery. I could have withdrawn and stayed in my shell; I could have given up when I couldn't do things, like lift both arms up in the air and hold them for longer than a minute – but I'd say to myself, *I'll try again tomorrow*, until I got it – it was definitely mind over matter for me, and the positive energy I created when I didn't achieve remained.

'Everything is energy and that's all there is to it. Match the frequency of the reality you want, and you cannot

help but get the reality. It can be no other way. This is not philosophy. This is physics.' – Albert Einstein

I was supported by Headway UK, a charity that supports people with brain injury, along with a psychologist and life coach. They helped me to focus on building myself up by using three simple methods – something we can all benefit from. The steps were originally taken from Professor John Evans, who showed that using positive psychology techniques could help people with brain injury or anyone going through some form of trauma.

In the latter days post-accident, I was taught to set three realistic goals and to focus on achieving them; so, at the start, the goals were things like going to the toilet without assistance, walking unaided, and being able to hold my hands up long enough to wash my hair (or lack of it). In time, I would set more goals and over time these goals became bigger and better. They got bigger and better because I eventually learnt to change the way I was seeing things. My inner self-critic was no longer giving me any doubts and I could see that by changing my thought process, things really were achievable. One of those BIGGER goals was to write a book one day in the foreseeable future. I used to tell my friends that I'd write a book to support others, and here I am!

I'm a true believer that if your idea – a dream or a goal – is bedded deep within you, you'll never escape it until you do it. I have learnt that you have to create your dreams, instead of chasing them. I am living proof that this method works – well, it did for me! Ok, I hear you; it's because I was always a positive person so it must just come easy to me, right? Wrong. I was actually quite negative pre-accident and was dealing with some horrible issues from some girls at school, I had very little confidence, and often had a murky outlook on life, and it was easier to fake a smile than it was not to. I guess back then I was silently coping with mental health issues and depression, which I highlight later in this book. My point here is that you don't have to be this amazing, perky person to become a positive thinker. I found that the more achievements I conquered, the happier I felt inside, and that over time created the positive attitude I had.

Being positive is a choice. You have to align yourself to it and practise all the time. Using positive psychology techniques prevents self-criticism and nurtures a set of personal strengths, competencies, and virtues. It doesn't matter how small these start out; it will create a new meaning and focus on life's outlook. One of the exercises I was assigned was to think of three good things that happened in my day. I would use a dictaphone to record these, and I would reflect on why they happened. It works because it stops you from thinking about what could go wrong or is already wrong and allows you to reflect on what is going right. The exercise helps us to focus on the positives, which gives us excitement and makes us feel good – and when we feel good, things tend to go right.

'Time has arrived for a science that seeks to understand positive emotion and strengths and offer us guideposts for the "good life" – new research into happiness shows that it can be lastingly increased.' – Desire A. Crevecoeur-MacPhail, PhD.

There was a time we – as in me, my doctors, and my family – didn't think I would be able to move my right hand again, let alone write. But let me be proof that the mind is an extraordinary thing – brain-damaged or not, anything is possible when you set your mind to it!

Did you watch *Game of Thrones*? Well, if so, you'll know who I mean when I discuss the Dragon Queen played by the beautiful Emilia Clarke. I bet you didn't know that she herself had brain surgery. Yep, whilst filming the second series of GOT. She is an absolute miracle – she went through brain surgery not just once, but twice, so let's be real here: you don't need me to tell you that she is an inspiration to us all. I don't know where she found her strength to go back to work and give her viewers (and we are talking 19.3 million viewers here) such a gripping series which amounted to eight seasons altogether, with the fans just not wanting it to end. Emilia had a subarachnoid haemorrhage – an uncommon stroke caused by a bleed on the surface of the brain, and now runs a charity called 'Same You' in support of brain injury victims. She shares her story on her website and has given numerous interviews to the media about her health. I admire her. We need people like her to take the stigma away from having a brain injury and help people get to grips with what brain injury is.

Emilia told the media that she found it hard to come to terms with having brain damage and stated:

I was suffering from a condition called aphasia – a consequence of the trauma my brain had suffered. Even when I was muttering nonsense, my mum did me the great kindness of ignoring it and tried to convince me that I was perfectly lucid. But I knew I was faltering. In my worst moments, I wanted to pull the plug. I asked the medical staff to let me die. My job – my entire dream of what my life would be – centred on language, on communication. Without that, I was lost.

I discuss throughout this book my own personal struggles from the loss of my identity. This doesn't come from a vain place. I know that it's not just how you look after you undergo brain surgery that matters, but it's an important factor when you're in your teens; in fact, it can be an important factor whatever age you are. Nevertheless, how we look is not everything; in truth, it's everything else – you lose a sense of yourself, such as your dignity, and that on its own was a minefield for me. Emilia reported in a separate news article that she felt *'deeply unattractive'* after undergoing brain surgery. She went on to say:

I know from personal experience that the impact of brain injury is shattering. Recovery is long-term and rehabilitation can be difficult to access. Brain injury can be an invisible illness and the subject is often taboo. In our society today – worldwide, in fact – we should be supporting people by allowing themselves to be open without fear, stigma or shame about their brain injury.

I can't even begin to tell you how fearful I felt when I was given the opportunity to write this book by Emma Mumford – when I sent her my book proposal, I held this light of positivity deep inside me, the hope, the need that she'd 'see me', the authentic me, and want to explore my ideas to help others on their long road to recovery, and to my sheer delight, she did just that. For those of you who don't know, Emma Mumford is a ray of sunshine; she is a certified Life Coach and Mentor, Law of Attraction Advanced Practitioner and Reiki Master. She has featured on *This Morning*, in *Women's Health* magazine, on the BBC and on the radio, to name a few, and she has a massive following. You can find Emma on Youtube and watch her videos that have really helped me over the years. When she said in one of her videos she was looking for authors who had a story that could inspire others, my intuition told me I had to get my book proposal to her! I didn't even have a proposal, but I knew that I had a story I wanted to share to help others. I sat up all night writing my proposal and sent it off in the early hours of the morning. I could not believe it when I was offered an interview over the phone! It sounds a bit cliché, but I knew that writing a book and having her mentorship was my intuitive calling.

When I started this book journey, I was fearful of opening up about the problems I have now, the fear of what others will think if they don't know me or, worst of all, if they know me but have no idea, and therefore start to treat me differently. Brain injury does carry a stigma with it – a rather big one at that; people literally have no idea how life-changing it can be. Like me much further on into my recovery, I found out just how invisible a condition it is, and even now, I am always justifying myself for the problems I have resulting from brain injury, especially with the aphasia and dysphasia difficulties I manage to hide so well from people in the outside world.

Support for Readers

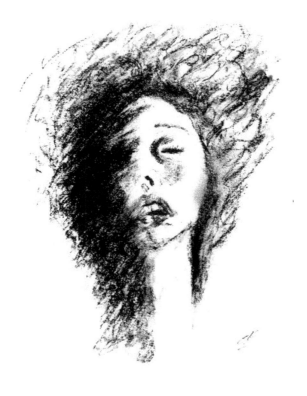

Illustrated by Steve Bromley

SameYou Charity:

https://www.sameyou.org

Watch Emilia Clarke on Youtube discussing brain injury:

https://youtube.be/VMkvZ16_Mvo

Positive Psychology

As I mentioned earlier in this chapter Positive Psychology was helpful in my recovery. Below are steps you can follow.

- Identify three goals to work towards.

- Work towards these goals slowly.

- Achieve goals one by one.

- Notice your confidence growing by achieving what you set out to achieve.

  Once you have achieved all three goals, increase them by one each time.

- Write down how you feel by achieving your goals, e.g. liberated, happy, anxious, and so on.

- Reflect on what is going right, and not what is wrong.

- Do not focus on the negatives; write them down and then throw them away.

- Gradually allow your goals to increase.

Notice how you feel about yourself; keep a journal on your positive feelings and thoughts.

Chapter Four
Now Let Me Tell You

'The new version of myself has very different needs than the old me.' – Kendra Partida

Now, let me tell you a little bit about brain injury, so as you read on you'll be able to notice the ways it affected me over the years. We can have different types of brain injury. Concussion is the most common type of brain injury and the least dangerous. It is reported that around 80% of all head injuries are from concussion, with the majority occurring in young people between ages five and sixteen. After minor brain injury comes moderate brain injury; this is an injury that causes anything between ten minutes and six hours of unconsciousness, and may cause amnesia (memory loss) for up to twenty-four hours after injury. People with this sort of injury are likely to be kept in hospital to be monitored to ensure there is no serious damage or secondary injuries. A person with this scale of injury may get headaches and fatigue, feel dizzy, and have poor memory. One issue here is that people expect their symptoms to disappear within a few days, but this is unlikely to happen, as it is typical for this sort of injury to last up to six months, if not longer. We really can underestimate our brains, and take them for granted, as we take most things for granted.

Then, of course, there is severe brain injury, when you are unconscious for over six hours. The person with this sort of injury, like me, needs to be hospitalised and is most likely to suffer permanent and life-changing disabilities. These can be cognitive, behavioural, or physical, and rehabilitation is required in order to minimise the severity as much as possible. As mentioned already, I received rehab not only from Headway but also from NHS clinicians. The extent of the disabilities sustained largely depends on how long the person is unconscious. For me, it was just short of two weeks. The longer that this is, the more likely that the person will suffer a serious deficit. The complexity of severe brain injuries means that every case is unique. It is possible for someone with a mild brain injury to make a limited recovery, just as it is possible for someone with a severe injury to make a complete recovery. Just like everything in life, nothing is straightforward, and we simply do not have the answers, and neither do the medical professionals. My neurosurgeons did not think I would walk or talk again, proving that even they cannot be one hundred percent sure of the outcome of any brain injury.

As we know, the brain controls everything that we do and stores our memories and personality, which is a big job for our little walnuts. However, it means that when the brain is injured the effects can range from minimal to extreme, and from physical defects to drastic changes in personality. This could be in a positive or in a negative way when we look at personality – and not everyone undergoes a personality transformation. Out of everything my family and friends said post-accident, the main thing was that I was still the Gem they all knew and loved.

This isn't always the case. On my trauma ward, there was a young man recovering from a motorbike accident. His newlywed wife, who'd just had a newborn, started to confide in my family, and she said her husband was a different man now, aggressive and argumentative. His wife told my family he used to be such a gentle soul, and she found it hard to support him the way he was post-accident. My parents told me that this patient had to have a security guard at the door of his private room, as he was a threat to other patients and to himself. We don't know if their marriage remains, or how his recovery was, but I only hope that he was given the support he needed so he could rebuild his life as a new father. If you just so happen to be reading this book, I hope that you made a good recovery.

The effects of brain injury fall into three main categories – cognitive, physical and behavioural. I hope you're sitting comfortably, with a cup of tea and something delicious to indulge in, because I am about to take you on a journey inside of our brains. I want to show how different functions of the brain are responsible for the workings of our own unique selves, and show how this can change for people with brain injuries – are you ready?

Firstly, let us discuss cognitive problems, where difficulty lies with memory, attention span, the ability to concentrate, to be able to perceive surroundings and to keep up with the speed at which information can be processed. Did you know that too much information can cause overload and can really tire the brain much quicker than is the case for someone who does not have a brain injury? Memory problems are a common symptom of brain injury because for a brain to process, store, and retrieve information many different areas of the brain must be used at once. If one or more of these areas is damaged, it will affect the person's memory. Post-traumatic amnesia (PTA), the medical term for memory loss, is when the injured person cannot remember what happened either before or after a traumatic brain injury. During this period, the person may find it difficult to recall or be unable to create new memories. The severity of the injury will determine the extent of the memory loss, meaning that it can range from the moments just before the accident, to a period of days, months, or even years. PTA is usually temporary, and, given time, memories can partially or, if we are lucky, fully return.

However, it is also possible that these memories will never be recovered, and this again depends on the exact case of the injury. In my case, I lost memories from my pre-accident self, memories of places and people, especially those of people who have passed away. I still have lows about this, but I remind myself through photographs, and I can visualise moments through the memories that others give me.

Moving on to our attention span and concentration, which are controlled by a part of the brain known as the frontal lobe – the part I had significant damage to.

There will be no surprises when I tell you that having a lowered attention span is common for someone who has suffered a head injury; in particular, the inability to multitask. Our modern lifestyles are quite badly affected when the ability to plan or follow simple instructions is compromised, and poor attention span can be further affected by factors such as stress, fatigue, and anxiety. This can lead to a vicious cycle, where a person is irritated by their inability to perform a simple task, which in turn makes them less capable of achieving it. Can I relate to this? Absolutely! In order to regain the ability to concentrate, it is necessary to 'relearn' how to do so through rehabilitation and distraction management – I talk about this shortly, because, at the start of my brain-injured life, following instructions was one of the biggest challenges I had to overcome.

If the brain is damaged it can cause perceptual difficulties where the brain is not interpreting the information from our senses correctly. There is a very wide range of problems that can result from perceptual difficulties; for example, for me, picking items up successfully, like a bag, a shoe, or a pen was really hard, partly because of my double vision but also because my hand-eye coordination was impaired. Despite being able to see them, I couldn't correctly determine the position in relation to my hand because of an issue with judging distances and spatial connections. It was a nightmare at the time, and I have a lot of empathy and understanding for those struggling with this.

When the brain is damaged it may cause reduced ability to process larger amounts of information in small spaces of time, usually due to changes in neural pathways. A useful analogy for this would be if you imagine a road system covering your normal journey to somewhere familiar was unexpectedly changed, it will take much longer to find your way than it would have before. This is an area I find very difficult; don't get me wrong, I still get to my destination, only a lot later than I had hoped. My friend Hannah will be having a giggle to herself just now, because I have circled a roundabout with her in my car more times than anyone should have to tolerate, or taken the wrong route – even though my wonderful, calm, Aussie-speaking Sat Nav said left, you can guarantee I took right! It doesn't really bother me now, and my friends have gotten very used to my directions being somewhat useless, so they know when they travel with me, they are in for an adventure!

Like myself, people struggling with slower information processing need others to speak more slowly, they may need to be given instructions several times before they fully understand them, and they may struggle to reply to questions in a 'normal' amount of time. My friends, family and partner get this; they add it to the quirks of being 'Gem' and we've all developed a good sense of humour over it – I mean, you have to, or else you'll allow your self-critic imposter to eat you up!

Just to make you aware, and on a very serious note now, this sort of symptom is described as the person being in constant 'information overload' and it is horrible – it's so unbelievably tough. Overload of information is an everyday occurrence for me. Because I look so 'fine', people just expect me to get it, and as a result, I always worry they'll think I'm stupid. But really, what I need is to take my time.

'The people that mind don't matter, and the people that matter don't mind.' – Dr. Seuss

As well as keeping our thoughts, memories, and personality, the brain also coordinates the subconscious physical processes that are essential to a healthy life such as breathing, hormonal balance, blood pressure regulation, the digestive system, and body temperature regulation. Without these functions, our bodies would not operate correctly and would cause an exceptional amount of day-to-day living difficulties. A severe brain injury can cause irreparable damage to the brain's ability to control these functions, so rehabilitative efforts shift from fixing the problems to learning how to cope with them.

Just because professionals say someone's ability to control subconscious physical processes is unlikely to return, this doesn't necessarily have to be the case. As I said earlier, they don't know for sure that things won't improve. Doctors told my family I would need 24/7 care, but we just don't know what is going to happen, especially when it comes to the brain.

A brain injury can sometimes 'rewire' a person's personality, causing their behaviour and emotional reactions to change. Exactly what is changed will depend upon which parts of the brain are injured. For example, the frontal lobe is the area of the brain that controls our personality and our impulsivity. If this area of the brain is damaged, it is possible that the person will

61

have reduced self-control or restraint and may not be able to moderate their emotions, resulting in irrational behaviour. The person may also go to the other extreme and have what seems to be an emotionless personality, known as 'flat affect'; this is something I can get when I am really fatigued, which is why I need to manage my sleep needs appropriately. It really isn't nice to be feeling that you 'should' have emotion but that you cannot seem to find it within yourself. It doesn't last long, but it's something people should be aware of. These types of symptoms are perhaps less obviously noticeable than physical problems, but they have a large impact on the injured person and their loved ones' lives.

A brain injury can sometimes change a way that the person feels or expresses their emotions. Damage to the frontal lobe may mean that they can lose the ability to regulate their emotions, and experience random mood swings that are unrelated to how they are truly feeling. Unpredictable outbreaks of laughter or crying are common, and they may feel like they are on an 'emotional roller-coaster'. They may have a reduced tolerance for stress and frustration, so even something as minor as having the television volume too loud or losing a set of keys can lead to an extreme verbal or physical outburst of upset. This is something I suffered from in the early days of my brain injury, but now I have fewer problems – well, unless my partner is snoring too loudly of course, but earplugs are a wonderful thing! I lose my keys ALL the time, BUT so do all my friends, which makes me feel a little comforted.

The ability to evaluate and adjust our personal behaviour to the circumstances around us is a complex skill, largely controlled by the brain's frontal lobe. Damage to this area can affect self-awareness, insight into the consequences of one's actions, and ability to show empathy or sensitivity. Those injured may also be unable to distinguish when they are being impolite or breaching social etiquette. Damage to the frontal lobe can cause a lack of motivation or spontaneity, though this is not the case for me. I was always motivated from day one of my recovery, and my best friends and partner will say I am spontaneous – I hear my sister whispering 'impulsive' out loud as she reads this – a little bit of impulsiveness doesn't do anyone any harm, now does it?!

Once the rehabilitation process starts, it is very common for someone to experience depression. This is especially the case towards the later stages of rehabilitation, as they realise the full extent of the problems caused by their injury and any permanent damage that they will have to cope with. It is worthwhile noting that depression is an important stage of mental recovery because it means that the person is aware of the reality of their situation. Only then can they begin to accept the situation and move forward. It is also perfectly normal for an injured person to suffer from anxiety, due to the loss of confidence they experience with situations and tasks that used to be commonplace. It is important that these difficult situations be faced head-on, with an attitude of independence, because if these fears are left to fester then the more likely they are to become a long-term problem – and us injured have enough problems to cope with, so don't let it become bigger than it has to be.

And finally, a person's sex drive can either increase or decrease. There are many physiological and psychological reasons for this, most of which are due to the hypothalamus (an important structure in the brain which controls hormone levels) being over- or under-active. This has really affected me (skip this paragraph, Dad!): I either have no desire for sexual contact whatsoever – this is especially so when I am fatigued – or ... well, the exact opposite (I don't want to be too graphic!) It's a bit like a roller-coaster – sometimes up and sometimes down, but things could be worse!

People with brain injuries can sometimes fall through the cracks of a system not set up to deal with their complex needs. As we have learnt, each brain injury is different for everyone, producing separate challenges for each individual. Neurosurgeons operate to save lives, but often patients get discharged into the care of GP's who may not notice subtle problems in intellectual function or changes in personality; people can get lost. I was extremely lucky to have been under the care umbrella of many professionals after my discharge. I'd have frequent visits to my neurologist which seemed to go on forever, I was on medicine for epilepsy, and had to be closely monitored.

FILM SPOILER ALERT – skip the next three paragraphs if you have not watched *Joker* and do not want spoilers. I have mentioned already in this book that I'm always letting the cat out of the bag, so I'm warning y'all now, stick with me or skip ahead!

I see you're sticking – that's great because I've enjoyed writing about this next bit; I'm guessing most of us have seen the film by Todd Phillips, *Joker*, right? Before I watched this film, a few people thought I'd struggle, which intrigued me and made me want to watch it even more. I took a lot from that film; it would be interesting to know what you all took from it. Of course, it's dark and mentally deep with an eerie tone throughout, but I couldn't help feeling some sympathy for the Joker. The start of the film shows Joaquin Phoenix playing Arthur – the Joker – struggling to make a living as a clown, and we can see from the start he has some obvious psychological issues. We learn about his disturbing childhood traumas, things we'd wish on no one. Naturally, this resulted in the Joker having conditions such as schizophrenia and personality disorders, amongst other neuro disorders.

Although in the film these conditions aren't specifically named, it's obvious he has issues with mental health and lifelong conditions that affect his brain. In one scene you can see him in fits of uncontrollable laughter, which he appears to get when he feels uncomfortable, embarrassed, or angry. In this scene, he's only really trying to make a young boy laugh and comes across as innocent. However, Joker comes across differently to the boy's mother and is seen as strange. He's confronted by the mother, who disgraces him, rolling her eyes, which makes Joker feel uncomfortable, unable to explain that he was doing no harm, causing him to laugh inappropriately and stand out to the public.

Joker goes on to show a card to explain his condition which states 'I have a brain injury.' The point of all this is that the film demonstrates the utter lack of understanding towards an individual such as Arthur – Joker – before he became the big bad mean Joker, before he was violent. At the beginning of the film, there is a scene where he was mugged by youths and beaten badly. Then we see his distrusting clown colleague offering him a gun for protection; naturally, he dismisses this offer, and we get the impression that he knows it is wrong.

Obviously, we won't come across the Joker on a bus, but we might come across someone who might be different: they might be swearing or shouting with no control over it or, like Joker, inappropriately laughing. Some people with brain injury can cry inappropriately, laugh, touch, or speak inappropriately, even though they are likely going through sheer upset on the inside. It doesn't happen to everyone and I'm extremely grateful that I have no trouble in this area, but I have spoken to people who have some of these problems in the aftermath of brain injury.

Again, as I am wanting to highlight in this chapter, conditions such as those discussed above are invisible, and I'm not just talking brain injury here; there are so many invisible conditions. I believe it's our duty as human beings to understand differences in individuals, especially today, which is why I say to you, dear readers, please be kind to others. We have absolutely no idea whatsoever why a person acts the way they do, so don't outwardly disapprove of them; inclusion is everything.

Coming to the end of this chapter, I feel it imperative to mention our impressive advances in medicine and neurosurgical techniques that have led to considerable increases in brain injury survival rates. This is exceptional, and I am so grateful for everyone working to help this happen. With the correct rehabilitation and support, survivors can make excellent progress in their physical recovery. Headway UK now provides a brain injury identity card – similar to Joker's. This is designed to help brain injury survivors explain their condition. A Headway service user stated that the card gives her reassurance and that if she was ever in a potential stressful situation, the card is invaluable in helping other people understand. I didn't have a card when I was younger as this wasn't on offer, but looking back, I would have rejected it because of the stigma it would carry. However, if I had my time back, I would use it.

Support for Readers

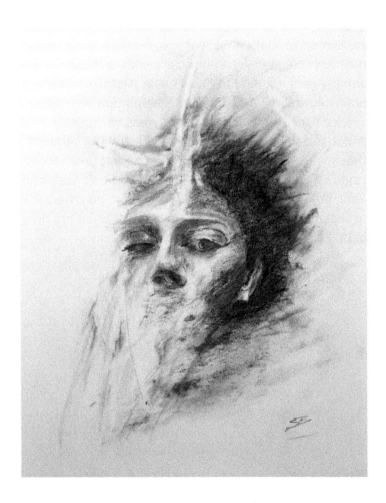

Illustrated by Steve Bromley

More information about your brain after injury:

https://www.headway.org.uk/about-brain-injury/
individuals/brain-injury-and-me/let-s-talk-about-sex/

https://psychcentral.com/news/2016/01/05/exploring-
long-term-effects-of-traumatic-brain-injury/97215.html

https://www.dummies.com/education/science/
anatomy/the-anatomy-of-the-human-brain/

- https://www.nhs.uk/conditions/severe-head-
injury/

Headway UK:

- Need to talk? Contact 0808 800 2244

- https://www.headway.org.uk/about-brain-
injury/individuals/brain-injury-and-me/my-
brain-injury-id-card/

Chapter Five
Baby Steps All the Way

'Whatever you do, don't congratulate yourself too much, or berate yourself either. Your choices are half chance. So are everybody else's.'
– Baz Luhrmann

Not long ago, my mum dug out some of my medical files to help me write this book. Along with them, she passed me a crinkled piece of paper that came out of an old dusty folder. I opened it up to find my name written in what appeared to be red crayon. At first, I thought my son (now five) had written it and I applauded him. I felt so proud of him, until Mum told me that it wasn't him and that I had written it when I had held a pencil for the first time in hospital.

Most people learn to hold a pencil in what is known as a 'dynamic tripod grip', something we learn when we are around six or seven years old. Younger children use what is known as an 'immature' or 'five-finger grip'. There is more to holding a pencil than we think – it takes fine motor skill, and this can be damaged in brain injury. For me, the parietal lobe, which is the part of the brain that plays an important role in our ability to read and write, had been damaged, so practising these skills regularly was vital for my recovery. Mum used to sit next to me on the ward and encourage me to practise holding a pencil, like I was back in preschool, and I am not going to lie, I felt pretty useless at the time. She would do this every day I was in rehab; she was single-handedly responsible for the strength I gradually built up in my right hand. So, when Mum told me that the writing I had found was written by me, well … I couldn't believe it; I just stood there staring at it in my hand. Then I had a vague flashback to sitting in bed on the ward with crayons in front of me and Mum pointing at something. Crayons, because they were easier to grip. I thought to myself as I passed the paper back to Mum, *Wow, was I really that impaired?* The answer was yes, I really was.

Now, I hope to help YOU give yourself some credit for all your achievements along the road to recovery, no matter how small they may seem to you, no matter what road of recovery you are on or whereabouts you are on the journey. Whatever traumatic event you have faced, you MUST allow yourself to appreciate the insignificant.

At the beginning of June 2002, I started to push myself to try to be a bit more independent, albeit I still needed plenty of help. I wanted to walk to the toilet, finally, because I didn't want to wear a catheter during the day. I had a walking frame and I managed to walk with Mum's help all the way to the toilet. This was a big accomplishment for me.

I hadn't seen myself since the morning of my accident. Mum was naturally worried about me looking in the mirror, as she thought it would be a shock. I can't remember this, but my family told me that I wasn't aware of what had happened to me. Looking back now, it makes me laugh when I envisage myself walking with my frame. I must have been slower than a tortoise or even a slug! Now, picture this: there I was, rocking my hospital gown that just about covered my bum, with my back arched, concentrating on my feet. I would drool like a dog and veer to one side as I walked, like I'd consumed one too many glasses of pinot! When I finally reached the toilet (and we are talking just a few feet) I peered into the mirror to see myself. I remember the mirror being steamed up from someone having showered in there. I didn't wipe the mirror – I don't know if that was because I didn't want to see a true reflection of myself. Possibly so. Mum said I put my hand on my head and looked at myself for a bit then just turned around to walk back. I didn't seem to care much about my appearance at all … at that stage of my recovery, at least. I remember that all I wanted to do was impress the medical team so they would let me go home, and the only way to do that was to practise walking.

There was excruciating pain in my head and face when I walked or moved my body. It was sore to touch, and I went for months without even washing my face. My eyebrows were out of control, and even when I did start to wash my face, I couldn't pluck my eyebrows because of the swelling. One eyebrow had been shaved off, and the other was so grown in, it looked like a slug (women would pay loads for eyebrows like it these days), so I looked rather unique, shall we say! Everyone involved in helping me through rehab required a lot of patience because, believe me, I didn't like help. I was determined to do everything by myself. Sometimes I would get so far then suddenly throw up because I was pushing myself too much. In fact, I wanted to conquer walking so much that I would try harder than I could cope with. I don't know why I did it to myself, as it was so painful to walk. I remember a feeling of intense tightness quickly followed by releases of fluid that would move slowly around my head and face. I can only really describe it like a lava lamp, where the lava moves up and down the tube in sluggish blobs. I could feel the fluid and see it move on my face; this was also noticeable to others.

When I was too fatigued, I was pushed around in a wheelchair, and boy did I love that! Andy would come and see me daily, and he'd take me for a ride. I say 'ride' because he would whizz me around the hospital corridors like he was Nigel Mansell, and when we reached a downhill section in the corridor, he'd let the wheelchair go! It sounds a bit crazy, but I needed this, we both needed it. I needed some normality and some light-hearted fun. Normally there wouldn't be anybody around as Andy would come to see me straight from work.

Andy was one of my sturdiest rocks during my recovery: he never failed to make me laugh, and later into my recovery, he was able to do the same for my family. I think it's important to have that one person who can take the mickey out of you, without ever being unkind. Andy would always be the first to tell me I was drooling. I had absolutely no idea I did this; the connection from my brain was damaged and I struggled with it for years after (but luckily, not on such a big scale). It happened when I concentrated, but fortunately, it's rare that I do it now! I didn't get embarrassed when Andy pointed this out though; I should have because he was the best looking, not to mention the nicest guy in high school, and it was young love or perhaps lust. We had a lovely connection, and mutual trust and respect. Having the support of someone like Andy, who wasn't family, was important. I believe he sped up my recovery by keeping my spirits high and helped me to feel beautiful – both inside and out.

You have to be kind to yourself and protect your wellbeing. You have to send yourself positive messages all the time when you are stuck on a loop in your hospital stay. Perhaps that's why I didn't mind so much about how I looked – because I felt so secure having such incredible people around me. Andy could have been shallow regarding my appearance, or he could have found the whole situation too much to cope with at eighteen years of age, but he didn't. My friend Sam reminded me that Andy would sometimes give me a gentle tap on the side, and I would literally fall sideways in slow motion because I had no balance whatsoever. Having 'half a head' – no bone flap – made me feel so much lighter on one side of my body, so it was easy to fall. We'd have a giggle, because you have to try to see the comedy in something so tragic, else not only might you have lost your identity, but your sense of humour too.

My physiotherapist Rebecca was lovely. Physiotherapy, however, was gruelling. I had to wear an eye patch when it came to mobility as I had horizontal diplopia and found it hard not to walk into things or to see an object when it was directly in front of me. I had no spatial awareness, and wearing a patch stopped me becoming a bruised peach! I found sessions with Rebecca unbelievably tiring. I started off with short bursts of ten to twenty minutes at my bed. I needed to do some physio from my bed to avoid further muscle waste, and to get the blood circulating around my body. I remember there being two types of exercises, called 'lower extremity' and 'upper extremity'. The upper extremity concentrated on my muscles from my waist up, and the lower were muscles below my waist. I remember finding the shoulder raise particularly difficult and it seemed to cause discomfort in my head. When we exercise, it is natural to make facial expressions. If something feels tough we might tense our jaw or squeeze our eyes shut. Have you ever watched a bodybuilder pick up heavy weights? Their facial expression says everything – you might even mimic them when you watch as you can almost feel the strain on their body. This explains the reason my head hurt so much. Our muscles are all connected and the strain on my face from the lightest of exercises was a big obstacle for me to overcome at the time – the pain was awful. Obviously, I had trouble remembering the exercises, given my short-term memory loss. My family was able to help with them, but I didn't enjoy doing them. I will go through these exercises in more depth in my self-help section as this may appeal to some of you. I did all my exercises when they were given to me – even though I didn't have much motivation to – because I knew it might hamper the speed of my recovery if I didn't, and I wanted to keep those bedsores at bay!

Rebecca was the one who helped me use my walking frame at the very start. She showed me how to get in and out of bed. Gran wrote in her notes that I had difficulty remembering how to do this, but with repetition I started to remember without any prompts. My mum and dad would often come to my physio sessions. When I started my sessions, I remember feeling more self-conscious of the way I looked, and how skinny I was. My parents said my spine stuck out so much, it reminded them of the Gollum, the fictional character from J.R.R Tolkien's legendarium.

I felt embarrassed when I couldn't do things, the simplest of things, like standing on one foot or balancing on a stability ball. I didn't realise it at the time, but I was in denial. I would see myself in the large mirrors they had on one wall and I started to notice that my appearance and my identity had changed quite significantly. I noticed my shaved head, the enormous dried blood scar, and how scrawny I looked. I felt unattractive and unrecognisable.

I have always been a people pleaser, and when I failed at completing a task set by Rebecca, I felt bad for her. I could see she was putting a lot into helping me – she went above and beyond for me, so why couldn't I do it? I felt so frustrated and irritated by my failures. The left side of my body was much weaker and occasionally the weakness in my hand and arm would defeat me. Rebecca got me doing some exercises, albeit very small, such as lifting my left arm, through mirror therapy. I found this extremely frustrating at the time, not to mention tiring.

I used to take my frustration out on my parents, mainly my dad. I was more ill-tempered and less tolerant in the early days after my accident. This is common for someone who has sustained a severe brain injury, and it gets better, it really does. The best way that I found to manage this was to keep a 'recovery journal'. If, like for me, writing more than a page is a struggle for you, a voice recorder is a good way to document your daily obstacles, such as feeling guilty for taking your frustration out on the people you love most. I mention guilt because this was such an imposter for me! I was constantly feeling down because I felt guilty for snapping at my family or Andy, for example, when I was unable to express myself correctly or when I knew a word but couldn't say it out loud. I know now that failures came hand in hand with fatigue, and with fatigue came poor concentration, and I was on this loop for quite some time!

I would like to explain a little bit more about mirror therapy. Although it wasn't overall helpful for me, I think I would have benefitted from it if I hadn't been in such disbelief and denial about my brain injury. Although I had a positive outlook the majority of the time I was in rehab, I didn't always have the patience to do certain tasks. Mirror therapy is a form of neuromuscular treatment, used to help many conditions to include brain injury, stroke, learning disabilities, depression, and anxiety, but it can also be helpful for other neuro conditions. Mirror therapy uses visual feedback to take advantage of the brain's plasticity (the muscle-building part of the brain) by using a mirror to trick the brain into thinking an area of the body works. It is a fascinating therapy to be aware of. It is suggested that you need to be able to have a good attention span for more than ten minutes.

Many people lose the use of their arm and hand after sustaining severe brain injury, and they may also experience spasticity – uncontrollable muscle tightness and stiffness which makes movement much harder. Brain injury interferes with your brain's ability to send messages to the nerves in your muscles. Therefore, I had difficulty in moving my right arm and hand in comparison to my left. In one of my physio sessions, I had to wear a restraining device on my better functional arm, which meant my affected hand and arm were required to do more repetitive tasks. This type of therapy is thought to increase brain plasticity (the ability to repair itself) and to regain function, in my case, of my hand. I cannot promise this will be the case for everyone in a similar situation to me, but your therapist will know the best techniques for you.

In the early days after my accident, once I had been moved to the trauma ward, I had a wonderful nurse looking after me. His name was Ben, and what a looker he was – if you've ever watched *Grey's Anatomy*, all I need to say is 'Dr Dreamy'- yep! So, before I started caring about my appearance, Ben used to wash me every day after breakfast. I remember he'd help me walk with my frame to the shower room – yep, there I'd go in that trendy blue gown that just about covered my bum. He was so kind and encouraging and would tell me things I needed to hear, things like, 'I saw you doing your exercises yesterday, you've really got good at them now, you'll be out of here before you know it,' and this gave me the motivation I needed. He must have been about thirty-five, my age now.

Later in my recovery, I didn't want Ben to shower me anymore. I became conscious of my body, and the high dose of morphine I was on made me hallucinate. I would often think that Ben had given me a kiss (cringe) in the mornings, to find out from my sister that he was just taking my blood pressure. I also used to hallucinate that he changed his hair colour and would sometimes turn evil, and I'd see him running up and down the wards. So, let's just say things got a little bit freaky, and I couldn't grasp what was real – it was horrible. It all gave my sister a good laugh; I remember saying to her one day, 'Oh here comes Dreamy,' and she said 'Gem, he is dreamy, and just think, he's wiped your bum.' Typical, that out of all the male nurses and assistants there, I get Dreamy and I learn he's not only been showering my skinny Gollum frame, but also been wiping my bum – great, just great! After Ben, my personal care was given by April, who was a game-changer for me. She made such a big difference to my confidence, and she'd bring books in for me that kept me going. I could always talk to her about my worries, and we'd often chat for longer than we should have at shower time. I still hallucinated, but not as frequently as before – probably because my meds were reduced over time.

If you didn't already know, morphine is an opiate, which means it is derived from opium. One of the symptoms of this drug is hallucinations, and boy did I have my fair share of them! Some are far too crazy even to tell you about – I don't think I'd ever live them down! The most frequently recurring one I had was an image of an elephant. I would see it all the time, even when I slept or while I had visitors. The hallucinations were mostly visual, but on a rare occasion I would be able to reach out and touch the elephant and feel its rough skin on mine. It felt so bizarre, yet so good: my mind was like a lotus opening and developing all these visualisations – I'd never had such epic feelings of anticipation of what was to come next. I guess I found it difficult to know what was real and what was imaginary. I also remember seeing a girl with a shaved head like mine, but she was more impaired than I was. She would come and stand by my bed and smile at me. Her stare was intense, and a little scary. She would always be there when I woke up from sleeping. I was thinking about it the other day – was she real or did I imagine her? I remember seeing her in both hospitals: Birmingham's Selly Oak Hospital, where I was taken in the air ambulance, and Birmingham Queen Elizabeth Hospital later in the year when I went to have my titanium plate put in. I think it was me – I was hallucinating and seeing myself, only I looked different in the face – my face was chubbier, which could have been the swelling. However, I can remember her laugh, so my hallucinations must have been auditory as well as visual and tactile.

We assume that hallucinations mainly involve seeing things that aren't there, but, in fact, hallucinations affect all of our senses, so there are lots of ways to hallucinate, as I have mentioned above, and it can be very scary for some people. Another type of hallucination I suffered from was a constant metallic taste in my mouth. I used to suck on mints to try to get the taste away, but it didn't make much of a difference. This is a type of delirium called 'gustatory hallucination' and it is very common in people with epilepsy, something I was medicated for.

Hallucinations after a brain injury can be terrifying when they happen. It's important to remember that these experiences are not real – they are just a result of neurons firing incorrectly. This also means that you shouldn't feel embarrassed or ashamed (easier said than done!) and you should not allow yourself to feel that you are crazy if you have a hallucination. Jo used to explain to me that parts of my brain were inflamed and that my hallucinations didn't reflect anything about my true self. With enough time, I regained control of my senses and my hallucinations stopped.

My rehabilitation continued and over time I got stronger and more able-bodied. I had support from school friends visiting me when they could, and I felt very loved by everyone. My school put together the biggest get-well card I had ever seen, and everyone rooted for me and wished me well. My oldest and very best friend, Jon, helped keep my spirits high. He would write me letters and keep me informed about what was going on at school. One of my other best friends, Emma, would also write to me: it was like having *OK* magazine hand-delivered to me in bed, only it was more *OK* magazine exclusive to Droitwich Spa High School!

We all go through difficult times. Having good friends when I was in and out of hospital was important for me to take those little baby steps along the road to recovery. My other friends, Sam and Rich, would bring me lots of treats – every time I saw them it was like having lucky dip and I loved it! It was so boring in hospital in the latter months when I was more able. Sam wanted to feed me up as I had lost so much weight, and she would bring me McDonald's – there's a bit of a McDonald's theme going on here! You'd think I'd never have wanted to see the glorious yellow 'M' ever again, but trust me when I say that you can only take so much hospital food! After my time in hospital, my dear friend Rich would carry a pillow around for me, because I needed it to travel in a car, but I'll get to that later because getting in a car took some time to crack!

Support for Readers

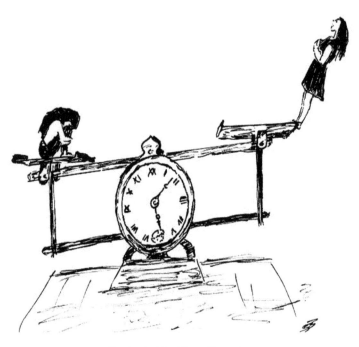

Illustrated by Steve Bromley

Charities that can help

'Brain injury can challenge every aspect of your life – walking, talking, and feeling, and the losses can be severe and permanent. It can mean losing both the life you once lived and the person you once were.' – Headway

UK-wide charity Headway works to improve life after brain injury. Call free on: 0808 800 2244 or email helpline@headway.org.uk

REMEMBER: THIS IS NOT JUST FOR THE VICTIM. THIS CHARITY HELPS FAMILY AND FRIENDS TOO. If you feel at a loss and are not sure how to support your loved one after they've sustained a brain injury, the staff at Headway are truly incredible people and want to help.

NHS physiotherapy exercises

If you just so happen to be reading this book while in hospital yourself, you may be interested in the exercises that my physiotherapist used with me. As I was in bed for such a long time, I one hundred percent believe that without practising these exercises my discharge wouldn't have happened at the time it did. Doing small bursts can help. I used to just do one of each exercise twice a day. Operate at the level you feel comfortable.

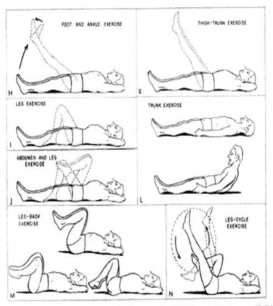

FIGURE 47.—Continued. H. Foot and ankle exercise. I. Leg exercise. J. Abdomen and leg exercise. K. Thigh-trunk exercise. L. Trunk exercise. M. Leg-back exercise. N. Leg-cycle exercise.

Mirror therapy

- https://www.flintrehab.com/2019/brain-injury-paralysis-recovery/

Hallucinations after brain injury

https://www.flintrehab.com/2019/hallucinations-after-head-injury/

Chapter Six
The Tapestry of Life

'Identity cannot be found or fabricated but emerges from within when one has the courage to let go.' – Doug Cooper

When I was about six years old, my mum recalls walking in on me playing with my Barbies in my bedroom. I had cut all the hair off one of them and had taken Mum's red lipstick from her make-up bag, covered my Barbie in this red lipstick and had basically ruined it, which of course Mum wasn't too happy about. I was never very good at looking after my toys, unlike my sister, who would have them all lined up looking immaculate! I guess you could say I was creative in my play and liked to think outside of the box. Mum asked why I had done that to my Barbie, and I replied, 'She was in a car crash, she had to go to the hospital.' Looking back now, that was a little strange. Was it a premonition? I have had a few premonitions happen to me throughout life. I believe that some people get them.

Regarding my future, I have always been quite intuitive. Obviously I didn't see everything the Universe had lined up for me, and by no means am I saying I am some sort of fortune-teller, however, I always knew that one day I would write a book about my experiences, and here I am, gratefully writing my book. I have always been into vision boards and I used these later in my recovery. I was sometimes silently angry inside, with echoing thoughts tormenting me, such as *Why me? What did I do to deserve this? I really hate being inside this person I no longer recognise*. I'd feel like this especially when I compared myself to others, which was a natural thing to do. For me, anger was counterproductive. For quite some time it prevented me from learning about my injuries, and I remained in denial for a long time, rejecting help.

As my rehab continued, I began to recognise improvements – I was becoming strong enough to complete the exercises my physio had set, I was sitting on a chair instead of spending all day in bed, I was writing more, and with Mum's help my handwriting started to improve. Although I wrote in a similar style to my five-year-old son, it didn't matter, because I was writing, and it felt good. My confidence was growing. My mum took six months off work to be with me, and Gran would come in during the times Mum needed to rest. Other family members took it in turns to be with me too.

By the end of July 2002, I was able to go home for a day at a time. I can't explain just how amazing I felt when I first heard this news. I was so excited to go home and see my bedroom. I was keen to get back so I could get more clothes, as I was always in tracksuits, which I hated (to this day, I still dislike them). I had lost my identity and that included my fashion style. I wanted to raid my own wardrobe to find some prettier, more colourful items of clothing to help me feel more like myself and more positive about the way I looked. I also wanted to have a bath, a relaxing, private bath!

My scar is about half an inch in width. It trails down, just off the middle of my skull. Back then, you'd have seen a powerful split – what I call 'half a head', hence the name of this book. My mum would help me with my personal needs, and wash over my scar. She had to be careful as my head was so sore and sensitive. I remember crying, it hurt so much; I remember Mum crying too. Like anyone, hair is hair and needs to be cleaned despite the length of it, but I hadn't had my head washed properly in months.

It was so nice to be home as all my family came to the house and we had a roast dinner. It was THE best roast dinner I had ever had – the goodness I was putting in my mouth as opposed to the plastic hospital food I had been consuming (and all those McDonald's). If you know me, you'll know that I have a BIG appetite and this roast dinner vanished within minutes! It felt for that short time at home like things were normal and nothing had changed. I was on a high, and I wanted to hold on to that feeling, but then I suddenly came back to reality and got a sinking feeling of anxiety: this was my life now and how I would manage would be up to me. I knew I had to see it through, and I knew that I was going to get through it; I just had to keep it switched on.

My stay in hospital was very bleak at times, and foggy too, but also a positive experience thanks to my incredible support system of family, Andy, friends, and the medical team. I was never on my own for long enough to plummet into a massive surge of depression – things were busy for me throughout my time there.

When I wasn't resting, I was doing physio or having visitors. My morale was mostly on an up. I'd often have low or angry days, when I'd get down about my new brain. Sometimes it seemed like it didn't behave, or I didn't know who I was anymore. I hated the person I could see in my reflection, but sometimes, I would forget and get lost in my old bubbly personality and feel like my old self again – it felt like I had two brains, or should I say, half my brain was on the up and the other half was on the down!

My dad would get me to look in a mirror and repeat after him, 'I am Gemma Bromley and I am beautiful' – I remember these times well. Although I would snap immaturely at him, refuse to say it, tell him it was stupid and be pretty horrid to him, I can see now why he did it. I do it to my son when he has self-doubt; it's a parent's duty – it's love. It was unfair of me, but I was struggling to cope with that new identity of mine, and I felt really messed up. It wasn't so much my appearance; it was that I had this imposter in my head. I had to get used to having a new brain, and that brain of mine had to get used to me.

When I was back home, I would go on regular walks with Mum in the week and with family at the weekend to build my strength. My family would take turns spending time with me, doing whatever was needed to help my recovery process. I would go out to the cinema with friends, but I found it hard to follow a full film back then, and I found it hard to sit still, but I made myself do it because I wanted to fit in. I loved going to see my sister at Bristol University. I went to stay with her on my own, which was the first big thing I did in terms of regaining my independence. I remember being there and feeling a little too messed up for it all – I felt like I was in a bubble. I literally had no confidence and I was paranoid about what people thought of my head. My sister was great; she knew I needed to rest and when it was just us, I was ok. But it was hard to have that confidence in front of people I didn't know. I used to wear hats, but my forehead was still dented, and I really struggled to look at myself. I was waiting to have my titanium plate inserted but I had to wait until all the fluid had settled.

I still had that lava sensation and, although people would think it was cool and unique, I despised it and I guess this is when my mental health began to suffer. I still received incredible support from family, Andy and friends – I was very lucky – but I couldn't make myself *like* myself. I started to be less positive and I felt completely lost. People used to say how far I had come, and what an inspiration I was to everyone, but it doesn't matter what people say to you when you are struggling with depression; you have to come out of that black hole on your own. Nobody can do it for you, even if they say the nicest things they can to lift your spirit. The nicer people were, the more guilty I felt. I knew I should have been feeling invincible, but I couldn't bring myself to feel anything but numbness – so let's just say life after hospital was the biggest challenge of all.

As I have already mentioned, friends were so important. They'd always be there for me if I needed them. This was especially true in my latter stages post-accident when I had returned home, and even a decade later from that, and even now, my friends have been my everything – you know who you are. They'd always offer help, but sometimes I wouldn't know how to respond to their kind offer. I mean, what could I ask of them without being a burden? However, I knew deep down that I wasn't a burden, but I remained the world's worst at accepting help.

There were a few things that they did help me with though, even without being aware of it. I formatted these into a list, as this might be helpful for someone else in a similar situation, or family members unsure of what to do when their loved one is discharged from hospital.

1. **Background noise:** In the early days, I couldn't cope with music playing in the background or having the volume of the television too high. I found it hard to tune out, and I found it harder to keep up with conversations. Keeping background noise like this low can be really helpful.

2. **A quiet space:** If I went to visit family for a get-together and there were people talking, kids running around and lots of background noise, my brain used to tire very easily. Although I loved to socialise, Jo would always send me off to a quiet space she'd prepared for me, normally for a power nap, away from the hustle! I used to accept her concerns when she'd notice I was tiring, even though I didn't feel it myself.

3. **Make it simple:** My family tried not to use too much imagery in conversations in the early days. My brain would naturally tire quicker in conversation, especially when they were too detailed. I didn't need people to talk slower (which I'd have found

patronising), but, brain-injured survivors need others to keep it simple at the very start of our recovery.

4. **Keep it positive:** Telling us we are doing great and highlighting our achievements helps us to feel positive and more likely to keep up the greatness!

5. **Have patience:** We will ask you to repeat yourself all the time, and we will forget information because our short-term memory is not as strong as it was. We might tell our friends that we'll be in touch but forget to call; please don't take this to heart, we can't help it! This isn't something that gets better, I am still like this now.

6. **Be the same you:** Don't treat us any differently; be exactly how you used to be with us – we need you to normalise things for us.

7. **Provide comfort:** I used to need to protect my head in the car; a helmet was too hard and sore to wear due to the swelling, but a soft item like a pillow was ideal to lean on whilst travelling. Not everyone will have pain in their head and loose fluid, but those who have had a craniotomy will need a few adjustments. It's much better that you offer them as opposed to us asking, because we don't want to be a burden.

8. **Be keen:** It's so liberating when you want to take us out, whether it be shopping, to the cinema or for a walk. It helps to normalise the situation and helps us feel part of a group. It creates inclusion. My friends were amazing at doing this.

9. **Acts of kindness:** When I went back to school, I had a boy ask me if he could carry my school bag to my classes. I will never forget this; I didn't take him up on the offer, but it was so nice to be offered the help.

10. **Awareness:** It's important to remember that we will get our words jumbled up all the time, shortly after hospital discharge and for many years later, and it helps if you fill in the blanks so we feel less inadequate. I admit this can still happen with me now.

This list will change as time goes on. Even though I am pretty much fully recovered, there are still some things you can take from the list which will make life that little bit easier!

I had occupational therapy after hospital, which was difficult at first as I had to do a lot of exercises that got me to use my brain – puzzles and word searches. I wasn't very good at them, especially in the beginning, but I started to improve and did so much better when I was not fatigued. I remember when I was in occupational therapy, I had to show that I could make a dinner for myself, so my task was to make some pasta. Simple, right? I mean, how easy is it to make pasta? Well, apparently not easy for someone with a brain injury. I started off putting the pasta to cook in a pan without any water, then I put the water in but forgot to use a timer, so my pasta was probably more mush than anything edible. Then I somehow managed to put the pasta sauce in the pan, only I hadn't drained the water. I felt completely useless – I used to be a good cook. I always used to cook at home and try things out, and I could certainly follow a recipe, so why couldn't I follow four simple instructions? I grew to dislike my occupational therapy sessions because they made me feel like I was impaired, and I wanted so badly to be normal again – but what was normal?

'There are over seven billion types of normal in this world.' – BUPA Mental Health Hub

I also had speech and language therapy. I suffered (and still do) from dysphasia. The best way I can explain this is if you can imagine you want to say a word, and it could be the simplest of words, and it's on the tip of your tongue, but you just can't say it out loud. It's basically a partial or sometimes complete impairment of ability to communicate resulting after brain injury. I still have to work to overcome dysphasia now at thirty-five years old. It's most difficult when I am in new company and the person isn't aware I have this condition. Meeting new people, going for job interviews, or being in confrontation with someone means I get more nervous and have to work extra hard to block dysphasia. It sometimes can be really overwhelming, and I get really frustrated, not to mention feeling the need to justify myself.

I got so much out of my speech and language therapy. It helped that my therapist was positive and liked to push me a little bit more each time I saw her. It wasn't just dysphasia I had to overcome; I had many other problems in relation to my brain injury. Voice volume and slurring, especially when I was fatigued, was a problem and I sometimes sounded like I was drunk – I still occasionally get this. I couldn't process conversations like I used to, and I was unable to organise my thoughts or focus on more than one task. I'd often lose my train of thought, and I would struggle to follow the rules of social conversations, for example, by interrupting. I also suffered with dysphagia, which is when swallowing is very difficult, and aphasia, which causes language and communications difficulties. With my therapist, I worked on specific goals. Together we'd strengthen my existing skills, through the use of word-finding tasks and problem-solving activities. We worked on multitasking during speech, which I found the hardest to do but finally made progress, for which I felt proud. My therapist got me to read and write and build on the work Mum had done with me in hospital. Not long after my sessions, I got into writing poetry. I even got one poem, 'The Neglected Map', published, so it must have helped. The poem describes how I felt with my injured brain, feelings of depression and hopelessness.

Writing poetry became a way of finding myself again. In despair, I would shut myself off from the world and write. It felt like a beautiful release of all the over-thinking I was doing, and it helped me to identify myself. I was keen to keep up writing, playing around with different words, so that my memory would improve and eventually my dysphasia would go. Writing is also a good way of coping with depression and it certainly kept me positive. I kept writing and still do. Not all of it would make sense, but it was cathartic and served a purpose, especially at that time in my life. Jotting down my experiences of hospital, rehab, school, friendships, family, and retraining my brain made me feel like both a young imaginative child and a wise old woman, who were coexisting in one brain.

Normal adolescence was almost alien to me. I felt I had to deal with so much more in comparison to my friends, but it was as if all this extra was going on in the background and that it was invisible to others. I think going through what I did made me realise that I was a mortal being and that my life would have an eventual end point, so I had to see the bigger picture and aim high. I guess I lost some of my childlike wonder in coming to terms with my near-death experience, and I realised that my life was limited. I felt lucky and was grateful for yet another chance in life. We don't have all the time in the world to accomplish the things we want. I stopped taking things for granted, people especially, when I realised no one has the gift of forever.

Alongside all my rehab, I had to repeat my year at school as I had missed so much. My psychology teacher used to come to my house and give me one-to-one lessons and did this without accepting any money. I struggled to break down information like I used to be able to do. I had to re-read things over and over and write them out until the information had sunk into my brain, and because I still only had short-term memory, learning was a challenge. I used a dictaphone, which I would recommend to anyone struggling with poor concentration and cognitive difficulties. To compound things, the normal one-hour lessons really tired my brain, and straight afterwards I needed to sleep. Despite this, I could always see a glimpse of light at the end of the tunnel. I had hope at my fingertips, and I remained positive.

I went back to school after Christmas, not long after I had my titanium plate inserted, and did half days. I felt liberated and more myself. To see my head whole again after having 'half a head' was beyond incredible: it was a miracle. It was tough for me to see my fellow school friends depart for university. I was excited for them all and wanted them to have the best experiences, but it just meant my friendships with some would change. They, too, needed to grow and move on to the next chapter of their lives. It was just hard to be left behind. Joining the year below me was scary – I knew some of the kids, but not very well. On my first day (and I remember it like it was yesterday), my lovely friend Alysia marched up to me with her big friendly smile and asked if I wanted to sit with her and her friends. She grabbed my bag and moved me over to them. Her friends were really welcoming and that was that; I found my place and it wasn't long until the new me belonged.

I used to hold so much anger, but I taught myself to remain positive, and learnt new strategies in order to create positive visions for myself. Back then, I had to work at being positive, but now, all these years later, friends old and new describe me as a very bubbly person, with a positive outlook on life. I think that anger is a weakness; it certainly was for me. Anger and resentfulness develop within when you feel vulnerable and do not value yourself. Over the years, I have found that I became less angry when I learnt how to love myself. Family support and friendships helped me with this. Instead of expressing anger towards myself and holding onto negative energy that used to suck the soul from out of me, I found solutions! I found the best way to manage negative and angry thoughts was to keep a journal of my thoughts and a gratitude journal of everything I was thankful for. Again, here I am telling you that writing can actually help you to mentally recover, as well as manage any anger you may be holding on to. My journals have helped me to release my thoughts and encouraged me to learn to let go.

My psychiatrist gave me a fantastic technique to use in order to avoid any self-doubt and negative thoughts. This tool was called 'TRUTH'. The TRUTH technique allows us to look within ourselves, to accept and trust our own feelings just as they are. TRUTH was devised by Tina Gilbertson in her book *Constructive Wallowing: How to Beat Bad Feelings by Letting Yourself Have Them.* TRUTH helped me to get past some difficult feelings and upset. So, instead of replaying the event over and over in my head, the TRUTH technique gave me a way to make my wallowing constructive. You cannot go wrong – there is no right way to do this technique, but the one thing you'll need is self-compassion.

So, what does it all mean? The 'T' in TRUTH invites us to *tell* ourselves the situation, and the 'R' stands for *recognising* our thoughts. 'U' asks us to *uncover* our self-critic, and 'T' wants us to *try* to understand ourselves. The 'H' of the technique is simply asking us to *have* the feeling we have after we have practised the TRUTH technique. By understanding our bad feelings, we allow ourselves to have them, and by the way – that's ok! The more comfortable we are with our own emotions, the better we will be; effectively it is a kind way of telling ourselves to get over it and move forwards. This technique is useful for brain injury survivors because we can spend too much time worrying about things, and can often over-analyse situations; it takes a lot of energy to fight with our feelings, so next time you find yourself wallowing, have a go at Tina Gilbertson's TRUTH technique.

'Writing down our negative thoughts will always eradicate the problem.' – Unknown

Support for Readers

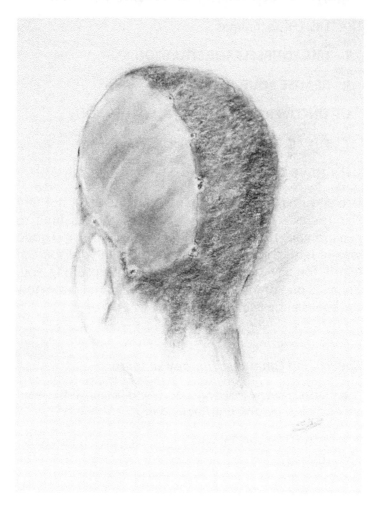

Illustrated by Steve Bromley

Constructive Wallowing by Tina Gilbertson

https://tinagilbertson.com/constructive-wallowing/

The 'TRUTH' Technique:

T - TELL YOURSELF THE SITUATION

R - REALISE YOUR THOUGHTS

U - UNCOVER THE SELF-CRITIC WITHIN YOU

T - TRY TO UNDERSTAND YOURSELF

H – HAVE THE FEELING

Use a journal to answer your truth; you might not find this exercise helps much at first, as it takes time to explore your thoughts. But I really do think it is a good way of letting bad feelings move through you. You can use it for any scenario that might be upsetting you. Below is one of my own examples to demonstrate how the tool can be used successfully.

Speech and Language Therapy support

- https://www.rcslt.org/speech-and-language-therapy/clinical-information/brain-injury

- https://www.brainline.org/topic/speech-language-therapy

Occupational Therapy support:

- https://www.brainline.org/article/occupational-therapy-brain-injury-recovery

Chapter Seven
Everything Happens for a Reason

'Bullies cause depression, depression causes suicide; are you a murderer?' – Anti-bullying quotes, Gecko & Fly

I have said from the start that everything happens for a reason, that life is a tapestry and it's already weaving a plan for you. Some people have to go through the rough to feel the smooth; this helps them to prepare for the next instalment that life throws at them – only they don't realise it at the time. In my story, this was certainly the case. I look back now and say to friends, 'You know what, if I hadn't gone through all that at school, I'd never have gotten through all this now'. There is a lot of truth in the saying 'What doesn't kill you only makes you stronger.'

Now let's transport back somewhat nineteen years. It was the year of the millennium, the year everyone went crazy for and celebrated in style, where hangovers lasted for weeks and weeks! I remember seeing Cliff Richard on stage and some other acts that couldn't have been very exciting as I don't remember, not that good old Cliff was anything to go by! I was incredibly happy because I was with my family – it was just me, Nicola, Mum, and Dad – and I remember feeling so grateful to have us all together on such a special occasion. That night was such a happy memory for me. After the show, I went to my good friend Jade's house and met up with some school friends. We carried on the celebration and I felt like I was in this bubble of pure happiness, with friends that appreciated me for who I was. School was going well for me, I was hitting my grades and studying hard, and I had a wonderful group of friends, both male and female. I've always had male friends growing up; I loved their laid-back approach to life which helped me to balance myself and avoid getting caught up in the dramas of a teenage girl. Even now my two friends Jon and Rich are still balancing me and helping me to grow, and of course, steering me clear of drama. Some people think that when you are romantically involved with someone, you can't have friends of the opposite sex, but for me, this is just not true. Friendship between men and women is not impossible, but it does require friendship goals that match – and luckily for me, they have helped me to find the important things I lost, like my smile, my hope, and my courage.

Life was good. I had (and I still do have) the most supportive and close-knit family I could ask for. I was always very close to my parents and could talk to them about everything ... well, almost everything. I have always had a remarkable friendship with my sister growing up. Sure, we had our moments of sibling 'love', shall we call it, but she put up with an annoying little sister following her every move. Even as teenagers, I would take her make-up without asking or wear her clothes and drive her around the bend at times, but I always aspired to be like her! There is an element of patience about my sister. She's possibly the kindest person you could meet, and she never has a bad word to say about anybody. I don't think I have ever heard her be unkind. She lets things go and lives in the present which is a hard thing to accomplish ... well, it was for me back in my teen days. There are three years between us, which we've never really noticed, and now we share some of the same friends. Nicola has always been my best friend. She has always supported me, not just in my recovery, but when I was younger, when school was a haunting experience for me. My intention for the next section of this chapter is to show that life is planned out for each of us, even the heart-breaking moments teach us, break us, grow us and show us that some things happen to help your future self be stronger, more resilient, and better equipped for worse things to come.

At high school, my group of friends and I took our fair share of bullying from a group of girls (we called them the 'hard lot'). They would target our group for one reason or another; we couldn't walk past them without them hurling abuse at us all or individually when we were alone. Naturally, our group rose above it and ignored them the best we could. There was absolutely no mirroring behaviour from us. Things gradually got worse, though. My friend Jade and I had some terrifying phone calls – somehow the girls had managed to get hold of our home telephone numbers.

I will never forget walking into the house one evening after a birthday meal out with family and discovering a message on the answerphone in which a girl shouted, 'Die, bitch.' At the age of fifteen, this was traumatic and hurtful, and my parents quickly became aware that I was getting bullied. Later the same week there was a phone call to the house again. The girl asked to speak to me, and my Dad just assumed it was one of my friends as she gave a false name. Taking the phone from Dad, I said 'Hello' and the girl (if you are reading this book, you know who you are) asked me straight away if I knew what my insides looked like, because I was going to find out. She went on to say my friend Jade was going to get a call as well and hung up with a roar of laughter in the background. I ran downstairs in tears, repeating Jade's name. I couldn't get my words out because I was so scared. My glorious meal out with family had suddenly been ruined by these girls.

Jade told me she remembered the calls very well, but said she was more worried about me because they told her they were going to kill me. My parents got in touch with Jade's parents and went into the school to sort it out the following day. The one thing I will say about telling the teachers is that it does not solve things. If anything, it makes it worse; well, it did for me. That's not to suggest you don't tell anybody if you are being bullied, whether you are a child or an adult, as it happens at any age. You could tell someone you trust or call the National Bullying Helpline (details in self-help section). They offer support and your call is one hundred percent confidential.

It may have seemed to onlookers that the problem had been resolved: everyone had been made to say sorry and things had moved on, but this was not the case. My friend Jade was and still is a very pretty girl and was popular. She now lives happily in Cyprus with her husband and two children. I think those types of girls – the 'hard lot' (and believe me, you will come across them in every high school) – target girls with something more about them, whether that is confidence, attractiveness, intelligence or quirkiness; girls who don't feel the need to pick on other people to get a laugh out of them. It makes me so angry just thinking about it. I think people can wrongly assume that a well-liked person is a big head, someone who loves themselves. In mine and Jade's case, that statement could not be further from the truth.

As far as I knew, things seemed to get better for Jade. She was always a bit tougher than me, and once you stick up to a bully, you gain a bit of respect. On the other hand, I got quite depressed, I hit rock bottom, and got into the frame of mind that I didn't want to be alive anymore. At that time, mental health wasn't recognised as much as it is now; to my knowledge, it wasn't highlighted as a 'thing' at all. I grew up without social media and my first phone was the size of a brick. And as for the internet … wow, that was a luxury! There are positive messages supporting mental health on social media nowadays and so much more help, which is great. Recently I was reading an article written by TV presenter and mental health podcaster Matt Johnson who talks about his battle with suicide and how he overcame this. It really resonated with me. He wrote, 'There are kids dying in the world, how dare you be depressed?' I think you can become ashamed of yourself for having feelings of suicide, guilt, and self-hate.

One day I told Mum I was poorly, and skipped school. Mum had no reason to think otherwise, as I put on a smile for everyone. I think some people at my school assumed that because I was popular in their eyes, I was fine – just like brain injury, suicidal thoughts cannot be seen. My parents thought things were ok, and why wouldn't they? I was a happy-go-lucky girl and appeared to be happy at school with many friends. I wrote a letter to my family and friends telling them I was sorry, that I loved them, but I couldn't take it anymore. I believed that their lives would be easier without all my burdens relating to bullying, and I raided the cupboards for pills. I was in a confused state, crying and scared; I'd backed myself into a dark and lonely corner of my mind, and at that time there was no snapping out of it. I felt that I couldn't continue my miserable school life, so I took an overdose and waited to die.

Now, let me tell you, when you choose to kill yourself you don't tell anyone. You might anticipate doing it for years, yet appear happy to those around you. You don't tell anyone because it's far too messy to even begin to explain, and where do you find the words? I should have spoken up and saved the upset I caused my family at the time. When you are being bullied, you think it'll go on forever; school seems like a lifetime. But it's not, I see that now. Hindsight is a beautiful thing. When you're called unkind names daily, when you read your name graffitied on the toilet doors and park benches, you start to believe you're not worthy and you lose your sense of reality. I had an amazing home life growing up, we had our family traditions and I was always myself – *'Gem'* – with them. I had inspiring role models to look up to and I was taught to treat everyone with respect. Trying to please everyone at school was a minefield and

I struggled with people's judgements when they did not know me.

After taking the overdose, I remember getting an awful migraine and blurred vision, and I was very sick – my body's way of rejecting the tablets. Even more messed up, I remember liking it. I wanted so badly to die. When my parents got home from work, they assumed I was still feeling poorly, just as I said I was earlier on that morning. They cared for me and kept checking on me. I didn't tell them what I had done; I stupidly thought I would still die – I thought my heart would just stop. I didn't really understand back then that it doesn't work that way. That evening my sister Nicola came in to see me for a chat about her day. Nicola was in sixth form at the time, which is where she met my brother-in-law Gaz. I liked having her in school with me, but we barely saw each other. Nicola would see me around and described me as happy with many friends. I confessed to her what I had done as I started to feel frightened and guilty.

It's a blur to me now but she told my parents instantly and I was taken to hospital. I was lucky, thanks to my sister. Taking an overdose can cause severe damage to your organs. I had no idea of the potential damage I had done which, in many cases, is not reversible. Even if you have your stomach pumped your vital organs are still very likely to shut down. You can die of liver failure and spend a few hours in agonising pain as, gradually, everything else stops working. People might think that overdosing on painkillers would be painless and easy, but the reality is very different. It is certainly NOT the answer to dealing with pain caused by other people's unkind treatment. You need to speak up, tell someone, because when you take that first step, things will get better, especially these days with so much information available on how to cope with bullying. I wish I had told my sister much sooner than I did. I was extremely lucky that I was ok.

I didn't tell my group of friends what had happened; it was just my family that knew, and some teachers were also informed. Life after that went back to normal. The bullying continued, but I was able to see past that after my scary experience and appreciate the lovely friends and family that I had around me. I still suffered from depression, but I didn't really understand it until I matured into my late teens. Thankfully, there is a lot more support out there for teenagers now in comparison to twenty years ago, and more school campaigns to prevent bullying. I know in some schools there are counsellors, and I think it is imperative that every high school has these. Teachers are on the front line, and whilst I think they do the best job they can, sadly, they have very little in the way of resources.

The scars left after being bullied fade over time, but the memories of it can last a lifetime, and it really depends on you as a person how you let that shape you. Alarmingly, the charity BeatBullying recorded 1,769 suicides of 15-19-year-olds between 2000 and 2008, which indicated that the total number of bullying-related adolescents' suicides may be in the hundreds. The charity found that every child suicide reported cited school as the main place of persecution. Nowadays, bullying is becoming a major problem on social media sites. BeatBullying reported that girls between the ages of ten and fifteen years old had the highest likelihood of suicide from bullying at school, tragically resulting in 65% of deaths.

Research carried out in 2016 suggested that online bullying is a contributing factor to many young people having thoughts of suicide. Over 200 schoolchildren die by suicide every year in the UK. We need everyone to be aware of the impact that online bullying can have on children and young people's mental health. I am so grateful there wasn't any social media when I was growing up, else perhaps my outcome could have looked somewhat different.

Bullying doesn't stop at school. There are bullies everywhere, especially in the workplace, and even in the home. Some of the bullies we knew at school have continued to bully and intimidate the people around them and may have used these techniques to climb the employment ladder to get to a position of authority. Bullies love to be in positions of authority, so they can carry on with their unpleasant ways. I know quite a few people who have experienced or are going through bullying in the workplace. The National Bullying Helpline also supports those experiencing bullying in the workplace. Recent studies have shown that workplace bullying is on the rise.

Research shows that nearly one-third of people in the UK have been bullied. Women (34%) are more likely to be bullied than men (23%). Shockingly, the highest prevalence of workplace bullying is among 40-59-year-olds, where 34% are affected. Sadly, in nearly three-quarters (72%) of cases, the bullying is carried out by a manager. Nearly one in three people who have been affected by workplace bullying have left their job. It doesn't surprise me one bit that bullying continues into our adult life. It's so sad that these people feel the need to put others down.

So, what can we do about it and how can we lower the suicide rate? The national charity Papyrus has put together a campaign called *#BedtimeStories,* aimed at school children, but I think it can also be helpful for an older age as well. This campaign hopes to unite against bullying and look at how we can create a safer environment for everyone involved. As I mention, in my own experience, online bullying was not a thing when I was growing up; this is also new for parents, carers, and teachers, so it can be confusing to know what the best steps are to take to help children cope.

Papyrus helps to limit the number of young people taking their own lives by breaking the stigma around suicide, and it provides young people and their communities with the ability to detect and respond to suicidal behaviour appropriately. The charity also helps with bullying in our adult lives in the workplace (see in the support section for further help).

'Remember, strong walls shake, but never collapse.' – Unknown

I am the person I am today as a result of growing from my experiences of bullying. Whilst I was receiving threats to my life, I was studying for my GCSEs. I started to skip school, so I could avoid the bullies, and my mental health, which I didn't understand back then, was suffering. I became very withdrawn and I ended up achieving lower grades than predicted. Obviously, my teachers didn't know what was going on, but after attempting to end my life, they soon discovered what was wrong and could see why my grades had suffered. I was lucky that the head of my sixth form – Mrs Moore – agreed that I could go on to further study after meeting with my parents to devise a plan. She was a wonderful support to me, and I will never forget that.

I think that going through such a traumatic experience at school helped me fight when I most needed it; every so often I wonder, if I'd not been the victim of bullying, would I have been such a fighter in the early days of my accident? It was like a mock-test to prepare me for what was to come! On return to school after my accident, I had missed so much work that it was necessary to stay back a year to catch up. I was still hungry for good grades and I studied so hard, getting extra tuition, and doing whatever I could to better myself. It was like my brain injury helped me to focus on being the very best I could – it showed me how precious life is and that I was saved twice from death, and that I really had no other option than to live life the very best I could. I ended up with As and Bs and was accepted into the university of my choice. For me, the lesson I learnt was that whatever setbacks you have, whatever trauma that haunts you, with determination you can achieve whatever you desire – after all, life is like a tapestry, and at some point, we all fall off a stitch!

'It takes a lot of strength to stay in the broken place, where you choose to gather yourself back up - piece by piece.' – Unknown

Support for Readers

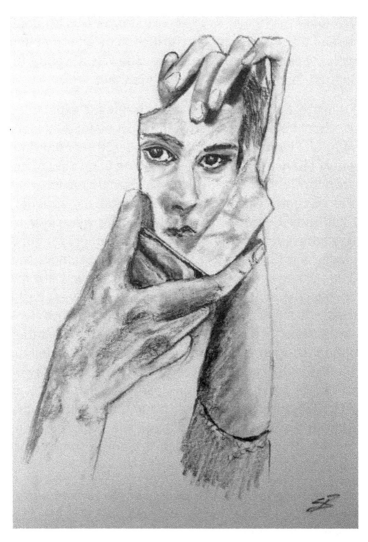

Illustrated by Steve Bromley

Below is some practical help on how to talk to someone if you feel depressed or want to end your life.

1. What do you want to happen?

You may need to talk to someone to help you understand how you're feeling, or you might want someone to give you some practical help. Have a think about this and about who would be the best person to speak to. A parent or a friend you trust.

2. Choose someone you feel safe and comfortable with.

If you can't talk to anyone or don't want to confide in anyone, call Bullying UK on 0808 800 2222. Their service is 100% confidential and you don't even have to give your name.

3. Think about what you want to say beforehand.

Would it be helpful to write a few things down? Or maybe you can draw something which might help you understand your feelings a little more. Use the pros and cons tool as discussed earlier. If you think about what you want to say beforehand, then you might feel more confident and prepared. Or maybe you just want to blurt it out, and that's okay, too. And if you find talking too tough, why not try writing a letter, or sending a WhatsApp, Snapchat or email? You could also speak to your GP.

4. Pick the right time and place.

You want someone to listen to you, so make sure you agree on a suitable time so that you can be sure you have their full attention.

5. Keep trying.

You deserve help and support – if you don't have a conversation about how you're feeling the first time you try, keep trying and whatever you do, never give up.

6. Write yourself a letter.

Sometimes it's difficult to talk directly to someone, even if you are close to that person. I can empathise with that. As it is so upsetting to talk about, the best way might be to write a letter to yourself, and after you have written it, read it back to yourself and see how you feel. It could help you feel more confident about approaching the topic. If you like, you could email or send the letter to the person that you want to tell – this will help the other person understand your position. However, sometimes the process of writing is all that matters, and the letter can be deleted or thrown away after it's been written.

Helpful numbers you can contact:

The Samaritans

Tel: 116 123

The Samaritans are available round the clock, every single day of the year. They provide a safe place for anyone struggling to cope, whoever they are, however they feel, whatever life has done to them.

Mind

Tel: 0300 123 3393

Mind offers thousands of callers confidential help on a range of mental health issues. Mind helps people take control of their mental health by providing high-quality information and advice, and by campaigning to promote and protect good mental health for everyone. They also provide a special legal service to the public, lawyers, and mental health workers.

Papyrus

Tel: 0800 068 4141

Provides support for anyone under thirty-five experiencing thoughts of suicide, or anyone concerned that a young person may be experiencing thoughts of suicide.

CALM (Campaign Against Living Miserably)

Tel: 0800 58 58 58

The Campaign Against Living Miserably (CALM) works to prevent male suicide and offers support services to any man who is struggling or in crisis.

'Never, never, never give up.' – Winston Churchill

The act of suicide is associated with giving up on life. By never giving up you are essentially building inner strength and resilience that nobody can take away. When giving up seems like the easiest option and the odds are stacked against you, always keep pushing and always keep going. By ignoring suicidal thoughts, they often accumulate. Sometimes life challenges us to keep going, even when we feel as though recovery is impossible. But I promise you, life can get better – trust me, I know.

Chapter Eight
What's Your Superpower?

'There is a superpower in all of us, we just need to have the courage to put on the cape.' – Superman

My little boy, who loves his superheroes, asked me, 'Mummy, do you have a superpower?' It's a good question, isn't it, and a very important one to a five-year-old. He told me that he is most like Spiderman (of course!) 'Well,' I said, nodding with a cheeky grin on my face, 'I would be invisible and then I'd be able to steal all of those peas you have left on your plate without you even noticing, in fact … wait there I will try and use my superpower just now.' He shrieked with excitement and soon shoved the peas down in one.

Most kids like to be inhumanly strong, fierce, scary but also a goodie who can save the world, a hero that we all love and adore, who can manipulate natural and cosmic forces or travel to the future. In every superhero comic, there is always that one power of invisibility, and of course, this power does in fact exist, just not in the obvious way.

Children usually stipulate that they should be able to alternate between being visible and invisible when suits, rather than permanently being invisible, because where would the fun be in that? There is a fascinating lure towards the primary notion of invisibility, as it gives us the opportunity to see things without influencing them. I mean, we already know how people act in our company, but we wonder what they might say to others when we are not there. I often think it would be nice to be a fly on the wall, so I guess if I was given a choice, I'd quite like to be Fly Man! Now he's a blast from the past!

Like with the power of invisibility, there is a fascinating lure for me to educate myself about invisible disability. Like with brain injury, other conditions such as Lyme disease, dyslexia and neurological conditions such as Tourette's, epilepsy, fibromyalgia, Still's disease, ME and autism to name a few, have one thing in common: we don't see them on the exterior, and this can create major isolation for the sufferers. For example, someone with Tourette's is more likely to be vulnerable to isolation in public places. I witnessed people move away from a man with Tourette's in a café. They made the heart-breaking choice of moving tables to get away from him and the vocal tics he clearly had no control over. Those people didn't appear to know about Tourette's, given their body language and behaviour. But, the man became more uncomfortable as a result of their actions. His volume grew louder, and his tics became more offensive.

There is a definite gap in society when it comes to invisible disabilities. I often hear about it on the news and on social media, but then there is always that one article you hear about that restores your faith in humanity. For example, I saw a photograph of a McDonald's worker helping a disabled person eat their food that did the rounds on social media, and of course, there are many more inspiring stories, videos and photos.

Sometimes I feel like I have my own superpowers that allow me to carry on and meet the demands of society, attain everything expected, albeit with pre-planning and a bit of impressive balancing. Let's just say that my life was turned completely upside down by my injury. I can accept my brain injury now. I will always have it: it won't get better. I have had to adjust in order to feed its demands. For example, when I am fatigued, I manage but I need to sleep as soon as possible. I often end up falling asleep with my little boy (probably before he does, most nights), and if I don't look after myself and care for my brain, my health can plummet. I have been known to end up in hospital because my immune system isn't very strong. When people are worn out and stressed, their immune system becomes weaker, and they become susceptible to illness. This happens to me if I don't manage myself well.

As discussed above, people with invisible disabilities don't want special treatment; rather, they want more awareness that they exist. I think it's important for people not to judge others. In my case, my short-term memory is such that, unless I see you regularly, I will forget your name, or call you the wrong name for ages, until you pluck up the courage to tell me, which happened to my friend Angela! Obviously, the penny does drop (eventually!) and I am utterly embarrassed and apologetic, but people tend not to mind. Then I have the need to explain my reasons and they often make a joke to cover my embarrassment, and say something like 'I actually prefer the name Amanda anyway', then I'll joke and say 'Well, you look like an Amanda, and at least I got the A of your name correct, so there is hope.' We can have a giggle and I feel at ease, but more importantly, I feel accepted. So, how nice are these people I've met? Those who don't even know what's going on with me but accept that I am pretty useless at name-recalling! Fortunately, I hit the jackpot with my group of friends in the playground at school drop-off.

Recently, my little boy started school and, it turns out, I seem to adopt tunnel vision when I do the school drop-off; I march my mini army of one through the gates and really that's my priority. I have hearing loss in my left ear – only 25% which is normally fine – but in crowds and busy areas, it is something I need to manage. Walking into the playground is a mammoth task for me, trying to socialise with other parents (because I like to socialise, and if you know me, you'll know I like to talk), keeping an eye on my child, listening to his needs, making sure he feels validated, whilst multitasking a conversation with Joe Bloggs next to me, discussing the weather, and so on. All this is something of a balancing act! I get fatigued by small interactions like this, but I love it all the same. I love that people think I am perfectly normal and look like a reasonably good mother. For me, the appeal of staying silent about my disability is somewhat liberating. If I say anything about my brain injury people often look at me with a flaky smile, as if I am having them on, until of course I say 'Yeah, so this part of my head is metal, would you like to feel it?' Do I do this to gain sympathy or reaction? Nope, I do it because I need a way of validating myself. I need to justify my sometimes airy-fairy comments and explain that I am not stupid. Did you know that we may only be able to hold four things in our conscious mind at any one time? For example, when we present phone numbers, we present them in groups of three and four, which helps us to remember the list. There is some controversy over this, but more and more it's been found from studies to be the limit. For someone with a brain injury, the filter mechanism that a healthy brain possesses to break down internal stimulus becomes broken and is unable to process information all at one time. After brain injury, the brain can only process one stimulus at a time. Recent research has concluded that background noise is disastrous for people with overstimulation. For example, the voice that someone wants to hear is one stimulus, and if you add in background noise it becomes two. Scientists discovered that in a brain injury victim, more brain cells work. There are more brain parts involved in activities than was the case before the brain injury. The difference can be seen with a head scan. Interestingly, brain parts that normally show little activity when performing an action are actively involved in the thinking process after brain injury. This requires many diversions and much energy. As a result, the reaction in a brain injury victim is often a bit slower. For every brain signal between brain cells, electricity is needed, which must be generated, and this takes energy, which can make the person very tired.

So, this takes me back to my situation where I appear rude to others because I have forgotten their name, or not heard a question they asked, or even have walked past them because I was concentrating on a different task. Straightaway, I explain my reasons (alongside an apology) and jump to explain 'I have a brain injury, half my head is metal ... FEEL MY PLATE,' in a sort of 'See, I'm not rude, I'm not lying, please like me, there's a reason I appeared rude,' sort of way. People are always fine about it, and usually I've blown up in my own mind with my worry about not pleasing others. I mentioned earlier on in the book that brain injury survivors are big worriers! We are paranoid about offending others. My good friend Rose jokily calls me Paranoid Paula! That moment of feeling guilt for not pleasing others is when staying silent about my invisible disability is no longer an option.

Naturally, when people are aware, one of the first things they want to know is what happened. When I tell them – and I have become good at doing this over the years – people are left astonished. I think that's a good thing. I don't want to be different, yet somehow, I am, because the only way I can justify my brain injury is to show my scar or get people to feel it. Why do I do that? Good question; I don't know why. I just feel I need to. My best friend Laura, my life rock, is constantly telling me off for justifying myself to people I don't even know that well. She's right, I shouldn't, but I do, because it makes people aware that you really can't judge a book by its cover, and it invites them to explore invisible disability more!

Having an invisible disability can be very isolating. I am lucky to have incredible people around me, who know my struggles, but I think that's part of the problem with some individuals: they suffer alone and haven't got a support system around them. I discuss support groups in the summary part of this chapter.

Despite having a wonderful support network around me, sometimes I still feel isolated with my injury. I need to work extra hard every day in order to stay connected because sometimes, especially with brain injury, becoming withdrawn is evident.

Today we are bridging the gap between disabled people and those able-bodied. There's a stigma when it comes to invisible disability. Some people don't believe it unless, like me, you have a wound to show. Others don't quite understand the seriousness of a disability and the effect it can have on your life. Disability is a very complex topic. If someone has a limb missing, their disability is without question, but for many others, it is not so straightforward

I'd like to bring to your attention some celebrities who live with hidden disabilities that you would never have known, which highlights my point of how invisible a disability really can be. First up and inspiringly true, Jessie J, famous singer and songwriter, has a genetic condition called Wolff-Parkinson-White syndrome, which causes an irregular heartbeat and shortness of breath, and at eighteen years old she had a stroke because of this. A stroke can result in brain injury which can be severe or minor, and I read that she struggles with fatigue. Jessie

J reported to the Daily Mail that she was very good at covering up her disability.

Next, one of my favourite actors and influencers, Morgan Freeman, who lives with fibromyalgia, an incurable condition not very well understood that causes chronic pain. Freeman developed fibromyalgia after a car accident in 2008. He went on to have many surgeries to repair his shattered bones, but he was left with nerve damage, which now disables his arm due to the chronic pain. I hadn't heard of this condition until I researched different hidden disabilities, but now the more I look the more people I realise suffer from it.

Avril Lavigne, singer and songwriter, opened up about living with Lyme disease caused by a tick bite, which means she lives with chronic fatigue syndrome. And the beautiful model Bella Hadid also suffers from Lyme disease.

I recently met a wonderful human being and fellow dog walker on the beach. We have been on a few walks together and she told me she lives with Lyme disease, so this is more common than I first thought. Interestingly, she told me that anxiety was a major disabling factor for her. Severe anxiety can also be seriously disabling. Actress Keira Knightly, who has dyslexia, openly talks about not being able to read when she was six years old and how she felt alienated as a result. She talks about how her brain works differently to other people's, but that it's ok, as people can excel at different things, and she jokes about how her spelling is awful. She says how hard it is to learn a script because the words jump around for her, and that early diagnosis is important. Other famous faces with dyslexia include Jennifer Anniston, Orlando Bloom, and Richard Branson. I admire these celebrities that hide their disabilities so well despite their famous lifestyles. I think as time goes on, more celebrities are speaking up about disabling conditions, and are saying it's ok, we have to support each other, we can all be an inclusive team.

'One billion people live with some kind of disability, and 74% of those do not use a wheelchair or any other aid that might signal their impairment to the outside world.' – According to the World Health Organisation

My beautiful friend Rose (the one who calls me Paranoid Paula), lives with dyslexia. I would never have known if she had not mentioned it. Rose has said that her dyslexia comes to play on a daily basis, but she has learnt many ways to compensate so that it doesn't usually present a big problem for her, and I am sure would agree she has come a long way from that thirteen-year-old girl trying to hide her disability through her school life. Globally, Dyslexia International (2017) suggests that between five and ten percent of the population experience dyslexia, which equates to around 700 million people worldwide. In my case, it is estimated that sixty-nine million individuals worldwide sustain a brain injury each year. The more we look at figures, the more accepting we can feel about our own condition, with the knowledge that we are not alone.

My friend Catriona lives with Still's disease. I knew I wanted to include her words in my book somehow, as they really resonated with me as I am sure they will with you. She said:

I am the face of a chronic illness. My illness is invisible to everyone but me. My health crashed three years ago. It felt like I woke up one morning and I couldn't recognise myself or my life anymore. It was terrifying. For a long time, my illness was an enemy, it was the thing that ruined my life. I would have given everything to go back to a time before I got sick. I spent a lot of time resenting my illness, but with time and healing, I was able to accept it as part of my life. I now recognise all the ways it has helped me to become who I am today. All I can say is that self-love is the greatest middle finger of all time. If you have someone in your life with chronic illness, believe them, support them and love them. They are dealing with more than you know.

Like so many, Catriona's illness is hidden; she's a hard-working nurse, mum, and wife, juggling life despite what lies behind the scenes. If you didn't already know, Still's disease is a disorder featuring inflammation; it is characterised by a high spiking fever, extreme fatigue, salmon-coloured rash that comes and goes, painful arthritis, weight loss, and nausea.

My seventeen-year-old self just wanted to get back to that 'normal' way of living. I made it to university and very much dismissed the help around me from therapists, rehabilitation experts, and life coaches. If I am entirely honest with myself, I disliked those professionals who had my best interests at heart. They made me feel different, and at that time I didn't want to feel different, so I shut them out and carried on. I shut out the world of brain injury and selfishly focused on being a teenager. Well, it won't come as a dramatic shock that I didn't last long at university; I was, after all, in complete denial that anything was wrong with me. I made some lovely friends and tried my best to keep up with the nightlife, but I found it hard to live the life others seemed to do so well at. I found it increasingly hard to combine both the level of work and social aspect of university – I struggled to party into the early hours of the morning and get up for my lectures – and that was when I realised I *was* different, and at that point, I realised just how much support and rehabilitation I still needed from my parents and those professionals I had dismissed so flippantly.

It wasn't long until I was back home with my family, trying to make the best of life. I spent some time in bed, as I became ill from pushing myself at university, and I lost a lot of weight. I tried my hand at a few things, hairdressing being one of them, but I failed at that too. I really didn't know what I wanted to do anymore, and teaching felt so far out of my grasp. I worked in a shop close to home for a while. I didn't mention my head injury to anyone, so working was difficult because I would often forget things, even just when working the tills or remembering codes. I ended up having to write memos everywhere. My manager at the time wasn't particularly understanding, but how could she be, not knowing about my brain injury.

The need to be the same as others, to conform to the majority was very appealing to me at that time: very different to the way I live my life now. As I worked one day in the shop, an old best friend who moved away when we were young came in. I'd always remembered her to be really nice, and she asked how I was doing – she'd heard about my accident and genuinely cared. I didn't think much about it when she left after a brief conversation, but I kept bumping into her! There was one time we met in a bar one night, and in the absence of a pen and paper, she wrote her number on my bag in eyeliner, which wiped off through the night. I began to forget about our encounter. BUT life works in mysterious ways, and although we don't ask for it, I believe the Universe has a plan for us all, and you meet certain people at exactly the time in life you need them most.

After a visit from one of my school friends, Holly, who went on to work with Virgin Atlantic giving beauty treatments to the likes of Kimberly Walsh, I felt encouraged to go to college and study beauty therapy. I coveted the experience Holly was having and admired her for it, so with a gentle push I found myself venturing on a new journey and one that really changed my life for the better. One week into my studies, a new girl started. From my view of the back of her head I knew I recognised her from somewhere, and it wasn't long until she turned around and gave me a smile, and I realised it was Laura – the girl I kept bumping into. So, of all the people in the world to be on my course, after so long, she was there. We pretty much picked up from where we left off and became close friends very quickly.

Laura took me under her wing. She was my rock at the time (still is) and my absolute saviour, and to this day I am proud to call her my very best friend. I have always said that there are friends, there is family, then there are friends that become family, and that is exactly how

I feel. I was struggling with everything I didn't recognise at the time: that I was depressed, feeling hopeless. I was at war with my brain injury and couldn't accept it. As time went on, Laura was able to 'see' my disability and the difficulties it brought to my daily life. She introduced me to her friends, who still are and always will be my treasures and, even though I don't see them much now, I know they're there. I believe in fate and I believe that if you invest selflessly into the world, the world will invest in you – I hit the jackpot with this lot.

I feel really lucky that old friendships found me. I lost touch with another best friend Emma as she went on to study nursing at university, and my other friend moved to Leicester; we connected again very randomly, and it was timed beautifully – just when I needed them most. Another good friend of mine I'd known from I was very young got in touch and she too came back into my life at the exact time I needed her. They all helped me to grow into my new identity and I am proud to have such incredible friends from school.

I will never forget sitting around a table with a list of professionals including my QC (Queen's Counsel), discussing my 'bleak' future. The meeting went something like this … *'She will need X amount of money when she has a baby because there's no way she could care for it on her own without a sleep-in nanny,'* and then some other professional piped up with *'She needs X amount of money because of her fatigue.'* So, there I was, feeling invisible, with my whole future being laid out in front of me, yet with no say. As you can imagine at nineteen years old, I hadn't thought about children,

I certainly hadn't thought about marriage (Andy and I had separated) and I had no idea what I wanted to do with my life, given I had recently failed at university.

I wanted to scream at them and tell them there was absolutely no way on this earth I will require help bringing up my child. It's crazy now when I analyse it: my mental health was in such a bad way, but nobody could see it because I am such a positive, get-on-with-it type of person and, if I was down, Laura would be the only person I'd let in. You can really fool the world around you being like that. If you smile, appear to be happy and hold a conversation, people don't have a clue that, really, you are dying inside. And at that very moment, sitting around that table with strangers predicting my future, anger doesn't really cover it. I was angry at everyone. I was angry for being saved, I was angry at my family and friends, but most of all I was angry at myself, the alien part of me, the metal part of me. The truth is these people had my best interests at heart. They were the first people to recognise that I had a hidden disability. They knew how hard it would be for me as I got older and they understood the impact my brain injury would have on my future. As I said previously, the Universe had a plan for me, and, twenty years down the line, I have brought up my incredible little boy without any help, and he is the reason I'm the determined mite I am today!

Support for Readers

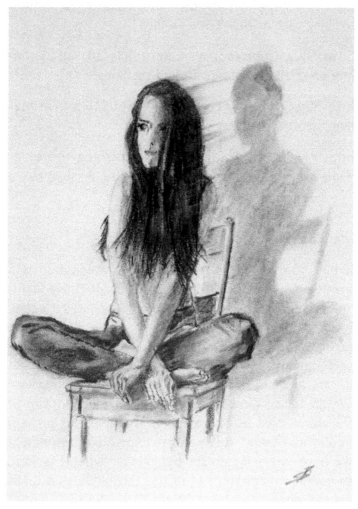

Illustrated by Steve Bromley

Be inspired by others

Here are a few sites I have visited that have helped me to feel more hopeful in my own circumstances in relation to living with an invisible disability.

https://www.bbc.com/worklife/article/20170605-the-hidden-challenges-of-invisible-disabilities

https://www.bustle.com/articles/160846-5-invisible-illnesses-that-are-very-real

https://www.psychologytoday.com/us/blog/the-wide-wide-world-psychology/201306/invisible-disabilities

Meditate

It has become widely accepted that meditation is a helpful way to reduce stress and anxiety, improve focus, and restore internal balance. Many people tell me they want to meditate but find it hard to begin. People who meditate and people who don't have one thing that is very much the same … their minds wander, they get fidgety, and they don't know what to do with themselves. We spend less time these days lying in a field looking at the clouds pass by, so slowing down and being present in our busy world is sometimes impossible. Essentially, we have lost self-care for our minds. When I wanted to learn to meditate, I used this technique that really helped me.

1. Find a quiet place and lie on your back. With your feet on the floor, bend your knees and allow them to lean in together.

2. Set a timer for the amount of time you can give to meditate and use a gentle alarm to alert you when that time is up. Start with two minutes.

3. Place your hands on your stomach, relax your body, and listen to your breath. Do not control your breathing – just breathe and observe.

4. Now bring in some visualisation. As you exhale, picture the sea, followed by a soft breaking wave on the sand. As you inhale, see it rolling back into the sea. With every inhale and exhale, watch the waves go in and out.

5. If your mind wanders, bring yourself back to the sound of your breathing and the image of the breaking waves; simply match the motion of the waves to your breath.

Travel Help

If you have a hidden disability and are struggling to manage it, help is available. The UK Government introduced the extension of the Blue Badge to people with less visible disabilities. This includes people with less obvious mobility conditions, autism, breathing or heart conditions, and other invisible disabilities. If you feel you would benefit from this, you can contact your local council to find out how you will be assessed. If, like me once upon a time, you think you'll never be able to drive, think again. There are many mobility aids that can help. I drive an automatic car which really helps with my cognitive thinking and helps me to focus better on the road.

Be guided by your disability

Make sure you tell your work about your hidden disability. They cannot discriminate against you, and it lifts a huge weight from your shoulders. I wish I had been more open about mine when I was younger. It wasn't until I moved to Scotland for work that I felt proud to say 'You know what, I have this brain injury and these are my downfalls because of it, BUT I assure you I am THE best candidate for this post because I am driven by these downfalls and work extra hard to overcome them.'

Learn to say no

I am the world's worst at this but, little by little, it's becoming an easier word to say. Saying no to all of the demands and requests, tugs and pulls on you is tough for anyone, let alone someone grieving from trauma, identity loss or losing a loved one. Saying no isn't just turning down a coffee date or a lunch with the girls … it can mean turning down extra work, no matter how much you need the money because, if it's going to cause stress, it's not worth it. Tune in with yourself, who you feel most yourself around, who really has your back. Tune in with the imperfect, messed-up you.

Some relationships are toxic, and the wrong people can drain your positive flow. Make sure you value yourself and when you do, the right people will follow.

Work

At work, your Human Resources (HR) team should inform you or train you about the needs of people with hidden disabilities. It is very likely you won't discover someone has a hidden disability until you get to know them better, when they may feel they are able to share more with you without fear of any judgment. Some people don't view their disability as an issue that they need to talk to HR about.

Chapter Nine
Feel the Fear and Do It Anyway

'The Universe is getting you back on your feet for the greatest comeback of your life. Are you ready?' – 15 Minute Manifestation, 2019

It took me a very long time to trust other drivers enough to get into their cars. I still get nervous to this day with a driver I haven't travelled with. This is the same for buses. I couldn't set foot on a bus for years after my accident. I don't know why; I just became over-anxious. I would wait for a bus, but start to panic, to the point where my whole body would sweat, the palms of my hands felt like they were pulsating and filled with cold sweats, and my heart would race like I was watching a thriller on television or when you get a sudden fright you weren't anticipating. Naturally, my body went into 'fight or flight mode'. Fight or flight mode is a feeling triggered by the amygdala, in the temporal lobes of the brain, and can occur in thirty milliseconds, which basically hijacks our regular thinking response, which can take 250 milliseconds. My experiences were, in fact, perfectly normal for someone who had been involved in a car crash involving a bus. I couldn't see it then, though, and allowed the feelings to imprison me in my own social life for quite some time. When we are faced with a life-threatening danger or we believe we could be in danger it makes sense for us to run away or, if that's not possible, to fight the danger. Feeling anxious and scared can trigger other bodily changes and make you feel very uncomfortable – this is a big factor for those suffering from post-trauma shock (PTS).

Here are a few other changes that may happen to you when you are in fight or flight mode.

- Racing thoughts – where you evaluate the danger and make quick decisions.

- Changes to vision – vision can change into tunnel vision where you can't focus on anything else.

- Dry mouth – this is part of the digestive system which shuts down on encountering dangerous or scary situations. This is because your energy is diverted towards the muscles instead.

- Racing heartbeat – this is because more blood is sent to the muscles in your body which will be needed for fight or flight and your heart is working like a trooper to maintain this.

- Cold hands – blood vessels contract and force blood towards major muscle groups.

- Dizziness – when we are in fight or flight mode, we create more oxygen and if we don't run it off, we can start to feel dizzy.

- Shallow breathing – quicker, more shallow breathing takes in more oxygen to control the muscles; this prepares the body to fight or run away (flight).

- Loss of bladder control – muscles in the bladder relax in response to certain stresses.

- Adrenaline overflow – this will signal to the rest of our body to get ready to respond to the danger.

- Sickness or stomach cramps – blood is diverted away from the digestive system which can cause our stomach to feel upset or even like we have butterflies due to nerves.

So, how do we let go of these feelings of anxiety and fear? In my case, I read the book *Feel the Fear and Do It Anyway,* by Susan Jeffers. This literally changed my mindset; however, it took me three full reads from front to back to follow the steps and make use of the tools provided in a way that benefited my own life. I wasn't ready to start some of the author's lessons straight away, but around eight months in, I got there. I made myself visualise what I wanted to achieve – getting on a bus, meeting friends, going for job interviews, and so on. I wanted my independence back and I wanted to let go. Susan Jeffers has helped millions of people overcome their fears with her profound advice, and her book helped me to take more control over my post-traumatic stress and feel empowered.

You could say fight or flight mode is similar to a panic attack. I told myself I wasn't destined to have panic attacks forever, but they do occasionally rear their ugly heads, even after all this time. They are different to manage now as a grown-up. Dealing with a panic attack is easier if you can find a way of controlling your breathing. Regulating your breathing will alleviate the attack's intensity. If you are on your own when you have a panic attack, it is the single most scary situation to be in, but don't let a panic attack get the better of you.

Nowadays, I can identify the triggers of a panic attack, and I am aware that one is coming on before the attack actually takes place. I found out over the years that, rather than fight the feelings I was having, I should try my hardest to adapt to them. I would visualise my feelings caused by the attack floating past me, without harming me, and I kept practising these visualisations until I became a pro at it. If I concentrated on my breathing techniques and remained calm, then, in time, the adrenaline would weaken and I could relax.

I used to suffer from panic attacks relating to many aspects of my accident, but as I grew older and experienced different lessons in life, I realised it was easy to pick up new triggers. Panic attacks can come from all sorts of different situations. I've found myself in unhealthy relationships in the past, and I can feel a panic attack coming on if that person gets in touch or is being difficult or manipulative towards me. I completed the Freedom Programme, designed for women as victims of domestic violence. This was hosted by Women's Aid, who were my angels in disguise. I received a great deal of help from them, and many tools I can use to help me.

As for getting back in a car, this was all down to the encouragement of four incredible people: my dad, who is the safest driver on the planet, Andy, and my friends Sam and Rich. As I mentioned before, they'd bring a pillow for me to lean my head against the passenger window. At this time, half of my skull was still missing and my brain had no protection. My titanium plate couldn't be inserted until the fluid settled. I felt safe doing this, and I pressed my head firmly into the pillow when we went over bumps and speed ramps, or even around corners, as it helped to cushion the pain I felt. I cannot even begin to tell you how painful fluid in your head feels. Going over a speed bump could feel like my whole face was going to burst; the pain in my mouth and my ears was excruciating, and my head throbbed.

I read another brilliant book, recommended by my dad, called *Who Moved My Cheese?*, by Dr Spencer Johnson, which I call one of my life's bibles. I continue to read it often to refresh my mindset if things start to look foggy. This book not only helped me to conquer my fear of public transport, but it helped me to go back to the learner's seat and drive a car myself. I did this after my occupational therapist assessed me to be capable of driving, though automatic cars only. *Who Moved My Cheese?* is a tale that helps us to unveil and reflect on the truths we have about ourselves.

The author wrote this book in an amusing and enlightening way. The cheese is, of course, a metaphor for what you desire in your life, for example, a better job, a pay rise, love, money, or literally anything you want. The maze is where you look for what you desire; this might be your hometown, your workplace or your friendship group, but the tricky thing is the cheese keeps moving! Basically, the characters in the book face unexpected changes in their search for the cheese. The book helps you to adapt quickly to change or to situations that you aren't comfortable with. If you choose to read this book and want it to help you, you have to think with an open mind – and it is not just for workaholics who wish to succeed, it can be related to any situation in life!

Even though I was already into vision boards or future boards – whatever you want to call them – I got more into them in my late twenties. Since then, I became a big fan of Emma Mumford and her Youtube channel. As mentioned earlier on in the book, Emma, along with That Guy's House publishers, has given me this incredible opportunity of writing this book. Emma gives some uplifting videos on vision boarding, and really makes them fun and easy to follow. I can wholeheartedly say that my boards have worked. A vision board is like speaking your dreams into reality, though obviously greedy ones won't get you anywhere! My visions were about recovery, education, and wellness. Now they are focused around the people I love, my business growth, my health, and spiritual growth.

At first, I didn't want to make one – at least subconsciously I didn't! But when I completed my first one I felt so liberated; it felt so freeing getting everything you hope for down to look at and manifest! The process was more of an art to me; it was soothing for the soul. Creating the board wasn't as hard as I had thought it would be – you don't have to accumulate years of pictures. Just as certain words inspire us or bring us joy, so can images. Creating vision boards has helped to keep me positive over the years.

I don't quite understand the karma behind a board; I see it more as a way to set out my intentions. Anyway, my point is that the things I hoped for, like driving, getting a safe car, having good friends, making the right career move, bagging that dream job, running that 10k, meeting my soulmate, creating my own business, and GETTING THAT BOOK DEAL have all been on my vision boards for years ... and yes, I have achieved every single one of them!

When I decided to learn to drive again, when I was twenty years old, it didn't actually take me long. I desperately wanted my independence. I had to go through numerous assessments by occupational therapy and neurologists. I was grilled for up to four hours, and had to undertake memory exercises, mathematical exercises, language exercises and some handheld brain teasers. This was a lot for my brain to cope with, and after the first hour, I was cognitively exhausted and was allowed short breaks. In occupational therapy, I was assessed on my reaction times, my ability to follow instructions, and I did a very long assessment that was marked on completion. I felt positive that I could get my driving licence. I visualised it, and I could almost feel the steering wheel, hear the sound of the road outside, even experience the gripping pain I still got in my head from going over bumps. It was all well within my reach and so, of course, it went on my vision board.

Not long after learning to drive, I was working as a teaching assistant at The Royal Grammar School Worcester. I absolutely loved the job. At that time, I still wanted to go into teaching, and I was really lucky to land a job through Laura's mum, who was the head teacher there at that time. Jane was, and still is, like a second mum to me. I know she will always be there for me, and she is someone I could go for coffee with, even if Laura wasn't there. She's known me nearly all of my life, and we have a lovely friendship. I admire Jane. She fought stage 4 cancer and could possibly be the most optimistic person I have ever met! She really helped me at various crossroads in my life. She even paid for my training in childcare.

Although I was happy working in the school, I wasn't fully settled. One day, I was looking on Google and an advert popped up for a degree course in rehabilitation studies for visual impairment. Straight away, I clicked on it, and to my absolute delight saw that it was taught at Birmingham City University. It felt right, and I even began to fill out the application there and then. It seemed to be a coincidence, but not long before I saw the advert, I'd popped this on my vision board!

Going to university as a mature student to study sight loss was the best decision I had made up to that point. It definitely felt right, and I felt like life was starting to come together. I remember questioning myself on how I would manage full-time education and working, especially considering the amount of fatigue I suffered, but I was determined to achieve this. I could see a clear vision and I knew I could do it.

I mentioned earlier that I moved to Edinburgh to bag my dream job. I knew that this particular job had my name written all over it, and I was entirely focused on getting it. I used affirmations daily – I'd tell myself I already had the job, long before it was mine, and I managed my nerves with mindfulness. It's very true what they say about mind over matter – I believe that if your mind is steady and well balanced, and you focus on the end result, the end result is sure to be yours. I practised interview techniques, rehearsed answers to questions I could be asked, and I made sure that I knew about absolutely every eye condition in the book! I even bought a 4D model of an eye to show my answers in more detail. As I was travelling back home on the train following the interview, I saw a little robin sitting on a bench nearby, and I knew something good was about to happen. Sure enough, I was offered the job, only a few hours after the interview. I was so grateful for the job offer and I knew that moving to Edinburgh would be the next positive adventure, and an adventure it truly has been!

So, if you were always intrigued by vision boards, or how to manifest your desires … give it a go, you'll be surprised by the results.

Support for Readers

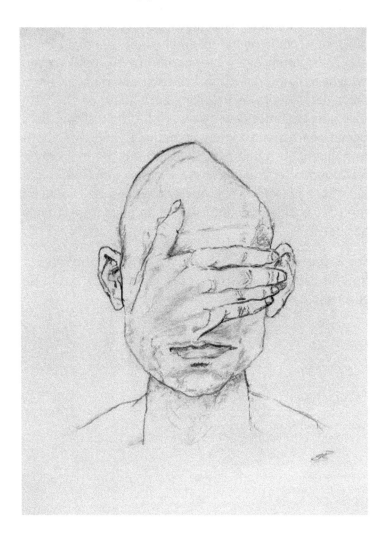

Illustrated by Steve Bromley

Vision boards

- Create a vision board for yourself, the now and the future of how you want life to look. This tool is one of the most powerful I have used and, yes, they really do work providing your energy is aligned with the positive energy you are able to create. Vision boards are an effective way to gain clarity on what you really want and to focus your intentions. Adding emotion to your vision board images will make it more effective in bringing your desires to life. I feel that the whole point of these is to set intentions, and if we can't see what that intention really looks like, we aren't going to be able to achieve it.

Manifestation:

- Visualise what you want to achieve, or even what is already happening, and watch your life start to change positively. Set positive affirmations such as 'No matter the challenge, I will persevere,' or 'I am confident that my feelings and thoughts are valid'. Affirmations can be written about anything and everything that you need to work on in your own personal circumstances. Here is a list which is associated with combating anxiety, which might inspire some ideas to get you started:

  o   I feel grounded and balanced.

  o   The panic I feel will not last.

  o   I am doing the best I can.

  o   I am enough.

149

o   I can be selfish on this occasion, because self-care is important.

o   I give myself permission to take a break.

o   Everything is going to be alright.

o   I am capable of anything I set my mind to.

o   I deserve good things.

o   I am strong.

o   I speak respectfully and kindly to myself.

o   I will continue to heal from past traumas.

o   Tomorrow is a new day, tomorrow is a fresh start.

Mindfulness

Mindfulness is a great tool to use when you begin to feel yourself wobble, when things are off-balance and you need some clarity on certain aspects of your life. I am studying a mindfulness course for children, mainly to use with my own child, but some of the strategies have worked well for me. Try this simple exercise: when you wake up in the morning, stay in bed and spend five minutes just looking around your bedroom. Notice the items in your room, the sounds you can hear from outside, the light peeping through the blinds. Then open your window and listen to the sounds more clearly – it could be birds chirping, rain hitting the window, dogs barking, cars engines, and so on. Next, make yourself a warm drink – this could be herbal tea or, if you're anything like me, a coffee. A good way – my only way – to set up my day!

Emma Mumford:

https://www.youtube.com/user/couponqueenemma

Books:

Who Moved My Cheese? by Dr Spencer Johnson

https://www.goodreads.com/book/show/4894.Who_Moved_My_Cheese_

Feel the Fear and Do It Anyway, by Susan Jeffers

https://blindhypnosis.com/feel-the-fear-and-do-it-anyway-pdf.html

Chapter Ten
Not the F Word

'Insomnia is a gross feeder, it will nourish itself on any kind of thinking, including thinking about not thinking.' – Clifton Fadiman

One of the conditions resulting after brain injury is fatigue. I learnt very quickly that if I didn't get sufficient sleep I may as well not even attempt to get through the following day without expecting it to be a challenge. This was especially the case for me in hospital, but it continued into my rehab, and even now in my adult life. Now, when we talk about fatigue, people presume you mean you're 'tired' – 'What's the matter with her? Man up, we all get tired!' But, unless you have had your brain vigorously shaken around like ice in a cocktail shaker, then we really cannot compare! For many brain injury survivors, a normal day is similar to when a friend might say 'I've been up through the night feeling ill,' or 'I was out last night, and drank too much wine' – the normal chat you'd expect to have in your social circle. But fatigue is very different, albeit fatigue is experienced by everyone at some stage in their lives.

For me, fatigue strikes after a period of physical or mental activity and serves as a warning to me that I need to rest. It's my reminder that I must rest in order to cope with the everyday challenges of being a good mother, going to work, keeping a household running smoothly, and so on. When it comes to normal fatigue, which happens to us all, it is time-limited and eased by rest. Pathological fatigue, on the other hand, the sort of fatigue I suffer, is directly a result of having a brain injury. This type of fatigue manifests somewhat significantly for most brain injury survivors, or those suffering other trauma related to the brain. Pathological fatigue is not alleviated with rest and is very likely to impact drastically on those people's lives, as it has on my own.

So, how do we get the dreaded F word in the first place? We know that it's a result of direct damage to the brain structures. Characteristics include sufferers requiring more effort to think or act. But what makes this fatigue and not something else? Studies have shown that there are many more diverse characteristics of fatigue, such as:

- Sleep difficulties

- Pain

- Cognitive difficulties

- Physical difficulties

- Hormonal difficulties

- Impaired sensations

- Reduced stamina

- Depression and anxiety

- Medical conditions

- Medication side effects.

I believe that all these factors can be managed adequately, perhaps not all at once, but certainly over the years, in order to gain back control in your life, as opposed to letting the fatigue control you. For me, to completely lose my sense of self in a life of fatigue was not going to be my happy ever after. It took me time and patience, support and acceptance (and don't get me wrong, it took me a good eight years) to learn the most valued lesson in life, which of course was to love myself again: the new me, the confused me, the forgetful me, the half of me, and the constantly tired me. If you can relate to this, or suffer from any of the above, or perhaps from conditions I have not mentioned, you too will learn to juggle your difficulties and accept the person you are, and those unique faults you so painfully judge yourself by. When you go easier on yourself, when you start to tune in to your body, you begin to feel empowered, and it is easier to manage the daily setbacks that fatigue creates for you, and see them as a challenge. And let's be honest, who doesn't love a challenge?

So, how do you distinguish ordinary tiredness from fatigue? We can't blame fatigue for all our problems, no matter how tempting that might be. Some days we might just be tired and feeling overwhelmed like anyone else might be. My suggestion is to keep a sleep journal. This will help you recognise when you are most fatigued and track the specific times of day when you feel at your worst. I suffer from migraines, speech problems, confusion (slower cognitive processing of information), and insomnia, and have learnt by writing this book that when I'm fatigued I overindulge in eating! But, more seriously, the big sign of fatigue for me is over-worrying about things that are superficial and bear no real significance, yet I can't help but worry.

Here are a few signs that have helped me understand if I am fatigued or just tired. If I am fatigued, I might feel ...

- more easily confused

- that speech and word-finding becomes a mammoth task

- that I cannot focus

- I'm suffering a migraine – not your average headache or a tension headache, but a headache that causes intense throbbing pain, nausea and sensitivity to light and sound (hemiplegic migraine). These uninvited migraines can also cause temporary weakness, numbness and tingling on one side of the body.

- fidgety legs, arms, feet and hands

- the start of a tic (for me, I tic more when I am fatigued, and usually in connection with something I am anxious about)

- sick and lightheaded

- withdrawn

- my eyesight is blurred (I get floaters that are temporarily present in my vision)

- irritable

- useless

- insomnia (sometimes we can get so fatigued, we become so restless that we cannot sleep)

- a loss of appetite

- like I want to overindulge in unhealthy foods.

It can be difficult to recognise these signs; this is likely due to the problems with sensory feedback to the brain, and this is where your journal comes in. It doesn't even have to be a sleep journal; it could be a health diary. I have more journals than you'd find in Waterstones! If you're not one who enjoys writing or if you have difficulties with writing, I recommend the Symple app, which helps you to track and study factors that influence how you feel. Symple was named the best healthy lifestyle app in 2019 by Healthline, and it has been positively reviewed by *Fox and Friends*, *Men's Health*, and *The Social*. Sadly, it is only available on Apple iPhones and iPads. I have an Android and I like to use an app called Journey, which is a motivational journal, which does much the same job and keeps me in touch with myself.

Factors you might identify in your journal could be repetitive mistakes you made at work at a certain time of the day, such as before lunch, when you are needing to feed your brain, or could be forgetting things you need for the day when you leave in the morning because you have too many tasks to attend to before you begin your commute to work. I found it helpful to ask close friends and family to keep note of signs that I might not notice, or I might not want to accept. Another good way of monitoring your wellbeing and fatigue is to score it on a rating scale of 1 to 10 as this will give you a better understanding of how different activities make you feel. The more equipped you are in managing how tired you are by keeping a record of the times you feel it can spiral, the better your lifestyle will become – trust me, you've got this.

Fatigue is a condition in its own right, and there is no cure. I found cognitive behavioural therapy (CBT) has helped me to become more aware of my brain injury and helped me to love myself for it. My therapist told me to carry a photo of myself around with me, and when I felt myself have a wobble, I was to look at the photo and remind myself how far I have come. I thought it was ridiculous at first – why would I want to keep the worst photo of myself close to me, let alone look at it? It took me a long time to make this exercise work for me. I found that one day, and I can't recall exactly when, everything my therapist had worked on with me somehow fitted into the empty space I had been holding on to for so long. Perhaps that was when I started on my spiritual journey, who knows?

If you are reading this only a short way into your journey living with brain injury, all these factors might seem quite overwhelming. You're not alone. However scary it may feel, starting to get help from early diagnosis is imperative. I stumbled on this quote a few years ago, and I think it's key to recovery:

'Success is the sum of small efforts, repeated day in day out. Take baby steps that you can add up to achieve incredible results.' – Unknown

CBT is an effective tool in many ways for aiding recovery. It challenges your personal beliefs. And for me, this wasn't just about accepting myself, but also the therapy corrected my misconceptions about sleep and taught me about sleep-promoting behaviours. The technique that really has helped me (and continues to do so) is called stimulus control therapy. This is where you learn to develop positive associations between sleep and your personal sleep environment, also known as 'sleep hygiene'. You learn little techniques that really can help, such as getting out of bed if you can't sleep, eating if you need to, avoiding screen time, and so on. Lying in bed getting frustrated because you cannot sleep creates a negative space in your bedroom and causes anxiety associated with sleep, which could become part of a routine if you don't control it. Sleep hygiene is basically the term used to describe good sleep habits. Considerable research has gone into developing a set of guidelines and scientific strategies which are designed to enhance good sleeping. You can download worksheets from the websites noted below.

Other recommendations to help with sleep are not to work in your bedroom or to use it as a space to do activity that can cause tension or stress. The goal is only to associate the bedroom with calmness, tranquillity, and relaxation, and to create a positive bedroom shrine of things that make you feel relaxed. I like my bedroom to be clutter-free. I need my cupboards and work surfaces to be clear and organised so that my mind feels clear, organised and clutter-free. I like to have inspiring quotes around me, artwork that means something to me hanging close by. I like to have a plant near to my pillows and some of the soy candles I hand-make. I also find it helpful to have a pillow spray. I use lavender to make my own and I've included the recipe below. Having certain plants in your sleeping space can confer many health benefits. Jasmine is the best for relaxation. Studies have shown that the scent from jasmine can reduce anxiety and improve sleep quality. Then there are snake plants, which are air purifiers, emitting oxygen at night to improve the air quality. One of my favourites, they are known to remove harmful chemicals from the air such as xylene, benzene, and formaldehyde, chemicals found in things like hairspray.

Another form of CBT which aids sleep hygiene is called paradoxical intention therapy. This aims to eliminate the anxiety associated with trying to fall asleep. Rather than trying to sleep, you challenge yourself to stay awake for as long as you can, thus diminishing the fear and worry of not being able to sleep. I have tried and tested this one at home, and I believe it will not fail you.

When I was in hospital, sleeping was difficult. I was on a noisy ward with elderly patients and I had to wear earplugs. But wearing these was so painful, especially with a swollen face, and often they didn't really even help. I found myself feeling really tired, and I had to sleep through the day to catch up, when things were surprisingly quieter. Sometimes I found listening to music helped, but I always remember using a fan by my bed, and the noise from the fan acted as white noise and I found it easier to sleep with this noise. I think, in fact, white noise is key for people suffering from sleep deprivation. In a similar way, I find a ticking clock restful, but not everyone is the same, so it's important to find the right sleep aids that work for you.

To recover as well as you can after any sort of trauma, you need to understand just how important sleep is. Many people have unrealistic expectations about how much sleep they need. Most of us feel sleep-deprived, the symptoms of which vary from person to person. When we experience long-term sleep loss, which can often happen after trauma, we can be more at risk of developing several chronic diseases. The unfortunate consequences of long-standing sleep deprivation include a greater chance of developing:

- obesity

- heart disease

- diabetes type 2

- stomach ulcers

- anxiety

- depression

- inflammatory bowel disease

- irritable bowel syndrome.

There are different stages of sleep that we go through, and these are fascinating to learn about.

Stage 1: This is when we first drift off to sleep – my favourite part of sleeping. We are in the shift from wakefulness to drifting, when we might feel completely relaxed and safe, and we allow ourselves to let go of the daily demands placed on us. We find ourselves falling into a wave of light sleep, where thoughts will emerge together at steady speed. It's a relaxing stage. The brain waves at this stage are known as alpha waves; as we drift further towards sleep the brain waves become even slower, called theta waves, but even then we are still in a very light sleep, and could easily be woken by even the smallest of noises.

Stage 2: This is very much like stage 1, but the body produces more rapid, rhythmic brain waves, called sleep spindles. Sleep spindles play an essential role in both sensory processing and long-term memory consolidation. These spindles are small bursts of activity immediately following muscle twitching. If you watch a dog sleeping, they'll go from steady sleep, where they remain still, to suddenly seeing their tail waggle and their feet twitching. My dog does this all the time, not to mention snores loudly when she is in this stage!

Stage 3: This is when very slow waves, called delta waves, start to emerge. Here, we are in a deep sleep and less likely to wake up to noises in our sleep environment. This stage is very important; it is where we top up on our beauty sleep! In this stage, we go into 'repair' mode. For some, it is common at this stage to wet the bed or to sleepwalk. This is especially familiar to me right now as I am currently helping my son learn to stay dry at night. Sleepwalking in brain injury survivors is common.

Stage 4: This is called rapid eye movement (REM). This name is derived from the frequent movement of the eyes in this stage. Adults spend 20% of their sleep in REM, as opposed to infants for whom it takes up 50% of their sleep. Sleep does not progress through all stages in order. After stage 1, 2 and 3, we can go back to stage 2, then we enter REM, and when the REM cycle has finished, we go back to stage 2 again. It's really fascinating when you think about it.

Hopefully, you're still awake and I haven't nodded off into the pages of this book! I hope you can all take pleasure in your next good night's sleep, well, after you've got your hands on a jasmine plant! I had to work with my rehab team in order to get a full understanding of the importance of sleep. I thought I was invincible, that I could carry on with late nights and little sleep – seven or so hours – but now I need no less than ten hours on an average night. Although I can get by on less, I get fluid on my head and this can become painful, especially when sleeping. It often wakes me up. That's just something I have got used to, my brain's way of communicating to me that I need to get more sleep. I think that anyone going through trauma, suffering with issues relating to mental health, or pretty much anybody that has been through or is going through hardship needs more sleep to help them recover and repair.

I was taught by Birmingham Brain Injury Centre how to manage fatigue, which has really helped me in my recovery over the years, and I still use their advice as my little 'brain bible' now. When I speak to people who have a brain injury or those who have been in touch with me looking for advice on other aspects of trauma, they often always start their message with 'It looks like you have your life together, how did you do it?' But these people are only just starting their recovery. My injury took place nearly twenty years ago. That's a very long time, and although the glory of social media never shows the 'true' you, as happy and positive that I am, I still have difficulties with the trauma associated with what happened, all this time on. It doesn't matter how you want to look at it, trauma is trauma and there is no running away from it. You have to face it and learn to manage it, else you can never move on, no matter how much you think you can.

I may be stating the obvious here but exercise in general, and planning and prioritising activities in particular to fit with your natural fluctuations in energy levels is extremely important. Something I have found harder to manage is diet. Maintaining a healthy diet is crucial for people who suffer from fatigue, and even to this day I can majorly fail on some days. This can wreak havoc for my daily routine, and it can sometimes spiral out of control. Why?

We need to feed our brain, but if we eat and drink the wrong stuff it won't give us the energy we rely on to do all the things we have to do. So, I drink absolutely loads of water – it keeps my brain 'clean', as I like to put it; I limit high fat and sugary foods; and I monitor the pattern of my eating, for example, the times of day I eat meals, to try to keep this as consistent as possible. Eating before 6 pm gives me a better level of energy for the evening. I have found that if I can incorporate a balanced diet that provides me with the appropriate amount of macro and micronutrients, my energy doesn't fluctuate too much. But it doesn't have to be difficult, expensive, or restrictive (I mean, if you know me, you'll know my love for chocolate, and I'd not give this up for a million pounds!)

Here are a few of my basic principles of eating better for more energy.

- Stock up on energy, don't limit your intake.

- Ensure adequate protein intake such as fish, chicken, dairy products, pulses, nuts, seeds, and meat alternatives like Quorn, tofu or soya.

- Eat plenty of fruit and vegetables – the recommended amount is at least five portions a day; each portion is eighty grams. These can include frozen, dried, canned, and juices as well as fresh produce. Pulses, beans, and lentils are included in this group.

- Eat a low-fat diet by cutting back on convenience and fast foods, butter, cream, mayonnaise, oil, crisps, and fried food. Don't get me wrong now, I love a takeaway and I don't cut these out, but I do limit myself to once a month.

- Try to resist the temptation to eat too many sugary/fatty foods – these include biscuits, cakes, chocolate, pastries, and ice cream.

- Drink two litres of water a day.

- Keep a food diary of what and when you eat every day.

- Take advantage of when your appetite is best.

- Drink lots of fluids.

- You can ask your GP to refer you to see a registered dietician.

Based on the five commonly accepted food groups – starchy food, protein, dairy products, fruit and vegetables, and fats – it is important to eat a variety of foods from within each of these groups to obtain a range of different nutrients.

Starchy food, or carbohydrates, form the basis of your diet, as they are an important source of energy. I don't know if you have tried the no carbs diet, but research suggests it's destined to fail in the long term. If you don't eat some carbohydrates your energy level will fall and if you suffer from fatigue, you're asking for a crash. I tried it, and it wasn't pretty. It takes us brain-injured folk a lot longer to rebalance, plus it will have a big effect on our cognitive functioning. Always get advice from a GP or dietician.

We know that protein is important for growth and maintenance of our body structure, and it's recommended that we aim for three portions a day. Nuts are the best and quickest protein snack that keeps energy levels up. Dairy products are just as important as a source of vitamins and minerals, for example, calcium and proteins. These sorts of foods can be high in saturated fats, things such as milk, cheese, yoghurt, and butter. You can get dairy alternatives; I have many healthy friends who use alternatives and their meals are delicious. When I was recovering at home, I would try to keep my cooking skills up. I would nearly always forget that I had food on the stove and my vegetables were so over cooked, I am surprised my family wanted to eat them! Overcooking vegetables will reduce their nutritional value so try to be better than I was in the kitchen and remember to set a timer.

Now for the best part – the fats, of course! Obviously, some fat is needed in your diet to be healthy, but it should be a limited number of servings per day in small amounts. Do we all stick to this? No, we don't, but I certainly learnt how to manage my energy levels better through what I eat, and I want to share this to help you.

Fats are a source of essential fatty acids like Omega 3 and 6, which cannot be made in our body naturally. They help reduce cholesterol levels. Something to highlight to people who suffer from fatigue is it is much easier sometimes to grab a quick fix or to overindulge in that packet of biscuits that tasted so good, but before you know it you've eaten the lot! You can stay on top of this by keeping a food diary, which can keep your diet balanced and your energy levels well maintained.

Support for Readers

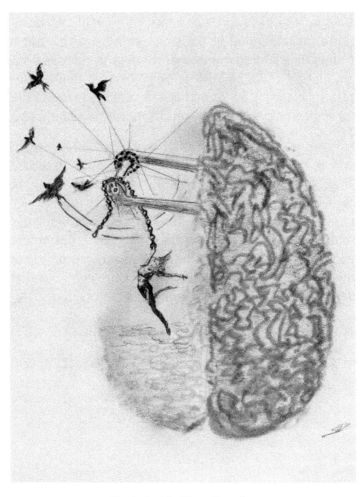

Illustrated by Steve Bromley

So, how can we make sure we get the best sleep? Below are some exercises which might be useful.

Sleep hygiene

- Set a schedule: Establish a regular sleep diary every day of the week. Don't sleep in for more than an hour, even on your days off.

- Don't force yourself to sleep: If you haven't fallen asleep after twenty minutes, get up and do something calming. Read a book, draw, or write in a journal. I always write my affirmations and things for which I am grateful that day. Do not use your phone or any other screen as they are too stimulating and will not help you to sleep.

- Avoid caffeine: Consuming caffeine, alcohol, or nicotine can affect both your ability to fall asleep and the quality of your sleep, even if they have been consumed earlier in the day. Can you believe that caffeine will stay in your body for up to twelve hours, and did you know that even decaf coffee contains some caffeine?!

- Take power naps: My advice, if you want to nap, is to take a power nap for no longer than twenty minutes; any longer and it'll make you feel groggy when you wake, consequently making you feel worse than you did before. And if you power nap, try to do it no later than 2 pm.

- Only use your bed for sleep: Your body needs to learn to associate your bed with sleep this way, when you lie down to sleep, you'll be relaxed and fall asleep easier. Using screen time is a big NO; it will stimulate your mind, and your bed will become a place for activity, which is quite the opposite to what you want to achieve.

- Sleep like a baby: It's important to sleep in a quiet, comfortable, and dark space. Using an eye mask, ear plugs, and white noise can really help you get that beauty sleep!

- Exercise and eat well: It's a no-brainer, really, but eating healthily and exercising throughout the day will result in longer, more restful sleep patterns.

- Don't go to bed hungry: When I was in rehab I was advised by my sleep hygienist that if I couldn't sleep, I should get up and drink some juice … some of you may be thinking that the natural sugars would make me more awake, but it does the opposite, especially if you are feeling a bit hungry. Going to bed hungry will not give you a good night's sleep.

- Freshen up your pillow: I make my own pillow spray from organic essential lavender oil, mixed with some rose water. You can buy pillow sprays, but I find they are very expensive and don't last for very long. I spray this onto my little boy's pillow too, and it helps him to sleep more soundly.

Useful apps for the phone

- Symple app for an iPhone
- Journey for an Android phone

170

Night-time snack tip

If you need a little snack because you feel hungry through the night, cucumber is one of the best things you can have! The phytochemicals in cucumber kill bacteria that cause bad breath, so not only are you eating a healthy snack to fill your tummy, you are also avoiding bad breath – win-win!

Useful links supporting sleep

https://msktc.org/tbi/factsheets/sleep-and-traumatic-brain-injury

https://www.acquiredbraininjury-education.scot.nhs.uk/impact-of-abi/sleep/

Chapter Eleven
When One Door Closes,
Another Opens

'Growth is painful. Change is painful. But nothing is as painful as staying stuck somewhere you don't belong.' – Unknown

The human spirit has the capacity to overcome almost anything. When we let go of the thought that we can't heal from something that has deeply wounded us, we open ourselves up to personal growth and positive change. Letting go means that we can make a start on rebuilding ourselves, albeit in our own unique way, that others may not understand, but as long as you do, and as long as you can see your vision become a reality, it doesn't matter if other people tell you that it's too soon, or that it's not possible.

From many years of experience, learning and understanding my brain injury, I can conclude that I am not, and was never, a 'problem' to be fixed. I used to have the attitude of 'I am not' or 'I can't' – these sentiments came from a place of self-criticism. When I changed my attitude and allowed myself more compassion in the areas that I wanted to change within myself, I created a place that was free of judgement, and for me that's when self-love overruled self-criticism. Granted, I was afraid that without prodding my self-critic voice, nothing would happen … but this was not the case, because change can and does happen, even without the nagging voice of 'I can't'. You see, the truth is that what my dad made me repeat all those years ago in the depths of my recovery, 'I am Gemma Bromley and I am beautiful,' was right all along. People going through life-changing trauma need to hear those words, they need to know that someone believes in them, someone can see their beauty within.

'My life can be described in one sentence: it didn't go to plan, but that's ok.' – Rachel Wolchin

You don't need me to tell you that by avoiding dealing with a past painful situation, it will only grow over time until it eventually becomes so big, you become lost. I have found that in order to heal you need to pass through the doorway of grief. Emotional wounds are sensitive, they're felt in the depths of your being, and it is hard to switch off. I knew that I needed to reflect on what I 'believed' had gone so frightfully wrong in my life, where it all started, and whether I could have avoided it. I gave myself permission to grieve, like we do when we lose a loved one. I was grieving my own personal loss of identity. I am in such a good place now, and I hope this gives you hope in your own circumstances, remembering that time really is a healer. I didn't do it alone, though – I needed patient people around me, and I owe a lot to my family and friends.

'A friend is someone who knows you as you are, understands where you have been, accepts what you have become and still supports you to grow.' – Unknown

Through my journey of coming to terms with my brain injury, I have learnt to let go of people who were not able to support me, especially in the early days. I think the key here is that these days we have the luxury of staying in touch with people from school through Facebook and other social media platforms. I speak to lots of old school friends this way, and I can cheer them on from afar. When I was in hospital, there wasn't that sort of connection for people, and it made my experience far lonelier than it would be now – we are talking well over a decade here! My good friend Emma used to write to me on a floppy disk! Imagine that! Then, of course, Windows Messenger came out and was all the craze. However, that little blue floppy disk was a memorable support system for me; it was my smartphone of the time, minus the apps and everything else attached. I'd say in this day and age, if you have a loved one going through something life-changing, check in with them, send them a message, call them up or write to them, because these small deeds might not seem like much to you, but to the person going through recovery, it means everything.

Although I lost some friendships along the way in my journey to now, this was ok. I guess sometimes a situation can be too big for some to handle, and without it being anybody's fault, it's just not meant to be. Of course, these friendships ended in the worst way possible, whereby nothing actually went wrong; we just stopped talking, they stopped keeping in touch, despite my efforts, and I got tired of being the one to initiate conversation so I just let them go. True friends – my seeds, I believe, can be counted on both hands! I believe that some friends leave to make room for others, better ones – the BIG 10. Despite that period of loss I went through, I realise how lucky I am to have kept the real treasures in my life.

For many of us, our healing takes shape only when we can un-become everything that no longer helps us to grow. For me, this included some friendships, relationships, and the idea of perfection of how my life was supposed to look pre-accident me, but now I live by this quote I stumbled on many moons ago …

'If you have to force it – relationships, friendships, yoga poses, perfect ponytails – let that shit go.' – Unknown

I have found that brain injury had a huge effect on my relationships with others. This was especially so in the early days with family and friends. I am grateful that my personality remained the same after my accident, and as a result I was able to keep most friendships, and even make new ones. I think this is because I am so inspired by other people, their stories, their successes, and their struggles. Having a brain injury has made me far more empathetic than I would have been without, and I must admit, a characteristic I love about myself. Writing this book has really challenged me to take a long look at myself and see how far I have come; I don't think I gave myself much credit until I started writing this book. It has given me the opportunity to explore brain injury further, and to learn about problems that others have, because their invisible disability is so uniquely different to mine.

It has also forced me to accept that even now, all this time later, I still carry an element of denial. This writing journey has helped me to meet other victims of trauma, and I am unbelievably grateful to have heard from these amazing people through the work I have been doing on my social media platforms. People have been reaching out to me for support in their own recovery and, knowing these people have really opened new doors for me, I am bursting with support and love for every one of them. One special lady that really stood out to me, who I am honoured to call a friend, is Rebekah from Northern Ireland, who is currently overcoming brain injury after being involved in a car accident. It was fascinating to hear her story. She always says how much I inspire her, yet really, it is quite the reverse. I asked Rebekah and her family if they minded me interviewing her for this book, they were happy for me to do so, in the hope that it will help others.

I find Rebekah particularly special because she is still on her road to recovery – three years post-accident, I have so much admiration for her, and as I go on to explain, you will see exactly why. Rebekah told me that she cannot remember anything about her accident, but she knew she was driving to the stables where she enjoyed riding horses. She told me that she will never be sure of what happened to cause her to lose control of her car but has always said she was trying to avoid a cat that was on the road. Rebekah's memory has been affected by her brain injury, and has lost around three years of her life, including some major life events, such as her graduation from university and being proposed to by her lovely supportive boyfriend. Naturally, this has been a source of sadness for Rebekah. She couldn't remember the first six months following her accident and even only intermittently thereafter. Firmer memories for Rebekah only commenced from about 2018. Rebekah suffered massive speech loss, her voice is now much deeper, and she cannot easily alter the pitch of her voice, which she feels makes her voice monotone compared to pre-accident. This is a particularly big loss for her, as she was studying and teaching drama before her accident. Like me, her rehabilitation programme involved a rehab unit, speech therapy, ongoing physiotherapy, and occupational therapy; this is ongoing for her.

Naturally, Rebekah's normal rhythms and layout of life feels lost for her; as you can see her recovery is still ongoing and it is taking her much longer to be able to do things such as walk and talk. I know she is still struggling with her body and has lost function in her left arm and leg. As I have said from the very beginning, brain injury is different and unique for everyone. Rebekah tells me she has taken a lot from my own recovery; she told me that recovery takes time, patience, and hard work. Rebekah and I have a support page for people with brain injury or family members who might need to talk; we give advice from our own personal experience and can signpost you to services that can help. We'd love to hear from you: details about our *Brain Dump* support group can be found in the resources section of this book.

Learning to bounce back is not easy. You might not be able to bounce back to the exact person you were. However, you are now even better than you think because you are unique, and really, this is quite the most refreshing feeling. I have found that I've learnt to enhance the unique little traits I have and like about myself over those that I do not like as much, BUT remembering to love EVERYTHING about myself, warts and all! We all play some sort of balancing act in life, whether we have a disability or not. Life is so busy these days, it's all so fast-paced and if we don't keep up, we begin to fall into the trap of self-destruct. However, my message to you is that life is not a race; we can only go at our own speed. Trust me when I say that if you can hold your head high and keep your eyes wide open to all the opportunities that are waiting for you in this magical world of ours, you will open new doors to the unknown, and who better to do this than YOU – after all, you've gotten this far.

Chapter Twelve
Hindsight is a Wonderful Thing

'Of all the words of mice and men, the saddest are "It might have been."' – Kurt Vonnegut

If you are reading this book, I presume you are looking for some support in your own circumstances. We all have times in our past which are memorable for being painful and difficult, times that we cannot bear to look back on because we haven't been able to gain closure on them for one reason or another. What if you could go back in time and show that past version of yourself the love and empathy you needed during those hard times? What if you could give your past self the advice you needed back then? I don't want to disappoint you; I mean, it's not like you can jump into Dr Emmett Brown's time machine and go back to what was. However, you can do the next best thing. Why not write to your past self? So, for a bit of fun, I have done just that. Writing a letter might sound like an ineffective way to heal your mental wounds, BUT it can be very therapeutic, and it's the way I wanted to end this book. I have found that hindsight is wonderful, but foresight is much better. I created my masterpiece (albeit abstract), and the creativity I found along the way allowed me to make mistakes. That was ok because it gave me the knowledge I needed to put into practice now.

This letter is unique to me, and it is authentically written from within. I would not change a thing about my accident; if someone said to me, they would give me my old brain back, I would tell them *no thanks*. It has taken a long time to find myself again, but I am now the happiest I have ever been. With my son by my side, my friends and family, my prince charming and the odd vision board ... anything is possible!

Dear seventeen-year-old me,

A lot can change in a decade or two ... in these tumultuous years you will see that all of your personal and professional upheaval was worth it, because you will look back and be grateful for every experience, good and bad, and you will become the very best version of yourself – you will be happier than you could ever imagine. You'll need to embrace these difficulties – you don't understand why, you're too immature to, but that's ok, just allow everything to slide off your shoulders.

I know you are in a very dark place just now; it doesn't seem that this will ever end – the pain you feel. I would be lying if I said your brain will miraculously bounce back to how it was. Just know that your future self still has struggle, but we have learnt to cope better. You'll be surprised to know that your new brain and you become friends, and you'll learn to deal with the horrible implications of your injury. You break away from the negative, emotionally stunted reality you are living just now, and you begin to heal from within.

Life really is a tapestry. Dad will say this to you, and when he does, you won't appreciate it; you can't really comprehend the value of those words. But, one day, you will value them – oh yes, you will. Dad will love the fact that he's right, and has been all along; he will be able to say that he told you so, and you'll tell him that nobody likes a gloater! You don't realise this yet, because you're in complete denial that your life as it once was will never be the same again; don't be scared of it, but try your best to embrace it. Just know that the errors made in life will lead us to that beautiful tapestry as promised – I can tell you now, it will resemble a jumbled up, messy masterpiece of mistakes, but also miracles. It will be priceless, and how glorious it will look, but you don't see that now, you can't – you're lost, and you have no idea who you are.

You don't have to push yourself to get back to school. The doctors predict you will lose a few years, and in the grand scheme of things, that's not so bad. YOU do not have to rush because you fear that you will be left behind. You don't have to worry that friends will forget you – they don't. You can take time out to think about what you really want to do – though you don't! Our impulsiveness never allows us to see the bigger picture.

You were right to fail the first time; failure makes us stronger. There is no shame that you need Mum and Dad right now. It might seem that everyone else appears to be independent, but we are different to everyone else; remind yourself that *it's not a race*. You really shouldn't punish your parents for wanting to help; they believe in you – in fact, right now they are your BIGGEST supporters AND you really need to give them a break, because after your first fail, you'll have many more.

By the time you are in your twenties, you'll start to see the bigger picture. Be patient, something we are not particularly good at with this brain injury of ours! Remember not to let other people guide your future. I get it, you want advice from those who care, and there is nothing wrong with seeking guidance, BUT don't forget to focus on what you really want. Use their words to help propel you into the future that you see yourself living, but don't ignore your intuition, because if there's one thing you will learn, and boy do you learn this the hard way, it's that your intuition will never fail you. There is a difference between guiding and controlling; make sure you know this, because not everyone who appears to care has your best interests at heart.

Hair is hair … it will grow back, so don't sweat the small things. You have it shaved off a few times, just after it has started to sprout back, and we lose our identity – yet again! BUT know that integrity is more important than hair growing back. Besides, you can hide it with a hat, and just so you know, those cringeworthy photos Dad took of you – aren't too bad after all! We are never happy with how we look – nobody is – but we eventually learn to be grateful for what we've got!

You plant *friendship seeds* that grow deeper, and wider. Their roots are tangled together with yours, holding hands, quietly nourishing each other to grow strong and happy. So, even in separation, they're connected and you can go for a year or more without seeing each other (and believe me, this will happen); don't worry though, they will always find you, just as they left you. You move to Scotland – YES you do – and friends will get married, they'll also get divorced, some re-marry, one painfully becomes a widow, but before that there was precious times and she made a beautiful baby; all of them make beautiful babies – even YOU!

YES, we have a boy, and after all that time, he is this reason we grew so strong. So, when you are told that you will need help having a baby when you are older – don't dwell on it. YOU CAN do it, and because of you he grows a heart as big as your own – which, by the way, is bigger than you think! You meet more *friendship seeds* in Scotland – lucky us. Yep – we find mummy friends, work friends, spiritual friends and some friggin' amazing neighbours – you meet your sisters from another mister, and you come to realise that if friends came with price tags attached, you'd never be able to afford such treasures. NEVER EVER underestimate the power of a chat with a friend.

Don't let your wonky walking knock your confidence – we eventually master the walking thing! Who am I kidding, we still manage to walk into things when our brain is frazzled, but we have a sense of humour! You will get words wrong most of the time, but you don't have to explain why to others or feel embarrassed – I'd like to see how they'd cope, if roles were reversed. It's tough to find confidence in your late teens, because at that age *we are all faking it until we make it*, by the time you are in your early thirties, you've enough life lessons under your belt to show your confidence, and this is sassy as hell!

You have a few heartbreaks along the way before you reach me (your future-self) and no, you don't end up with Andy, but he's shown you what a gentleman is, and that is why you should never settle for anything less. Alas, you do … and this will teach you and grow you more than you think is possible. You learn the skills to let go of that person/people who have taken so much out of your life, and from your time. Your best friend Laura (yes, Laura), your childhood seed finds you again, just when all your hope feels lost. She was right, you do meet your prince charming muuuuuuuuch later on in life, and after finally letting him in, you find that he's the most profoundly good person you have ever met, and you'll never have to question his good intentions.

Over time you will learn that playing small will not serve the world. There is no success in shrinking so that other people will not feel insecure around you. Remember, we did this when we were bullied at school – we got shrunk. You're probably too trusting, and naïve, you tend to see the good in the bad people, but we know that not everything is as it seems, and this goes for yourself!

So, dear seventeen-year-old me, know this: all the people you meet in life and the success and downfalls you experience help to become the future-you, the fabulous you! All the bad experiences can be learned from; in fact, they are probably the most poignant and important life lessons. If someone hurts you, ridicules you, betrays you, or treats you unkindly – forgive them; you don't need to carry that around in your life. Know that nothing happens by chance – illness, injury, love, lost moments of true greatness and sheer stupidity all occur to test your limits. You find your purpose in life, which you knew all along was to help others, and that is exactly what you go on to do. You own and grow a business in-between and you work harder than you've ever worked – but you do it, because that's how we do things – we work hard! Annnnnd lastly, that book you keep telling your friends you'll write one day – WE do it, WE smash it, and WE can thank our brain injury for that!

Now, I know that we love a quote, so I will leave you with this:

'Somewhere there is a past you, overflowing with so much pride looking at how far you've come.' – Jess Rachel Sharp

Seventeen-year-old me, NEVER give up.

Love, me (your future-self)

If you can take anything from this book, I hope it'll be that you should never underestimate the power of the human spirit. I was once in close proximity of death, so close I was practically knocking on its door. Just remember that when life gives you lemons, you have the choice to make the BEST lemonade on the market or you could let them go mouldy – it's your call. Nineteen years ago, my doctors told my family to prepare themselves, they told them they should say goodbye. BUT against all the odds, my human spirit helped me to overcome adversity – and boy did I make lemonade! I found the strength within to flourish, so I could create wings and fly, just as my sister said at the very beginning. You too can break free of your cocoon, and have faith that whatever hardship you face, whatever trauma you endure, your human spirit will help you fly – and make lemonade!

All my love,

Gemma x

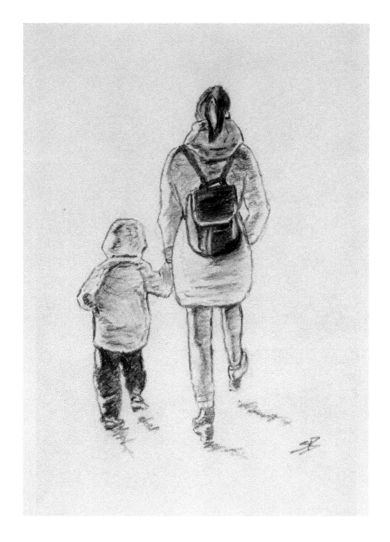

Illustrated by Steve Bromley

**The End
(or just the beginning)**

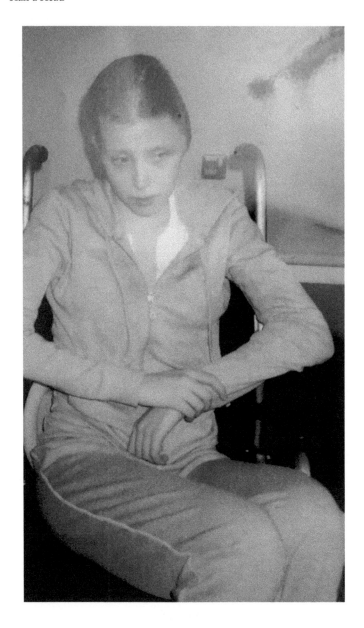

Rehab 2002

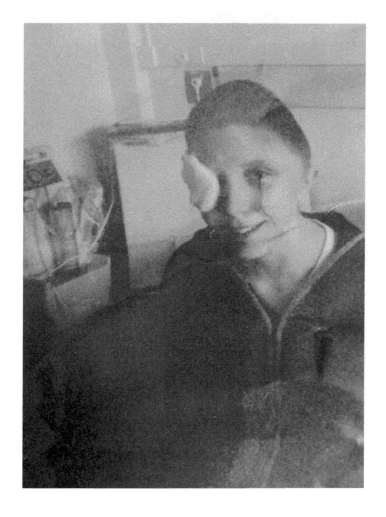

Rehab 2002

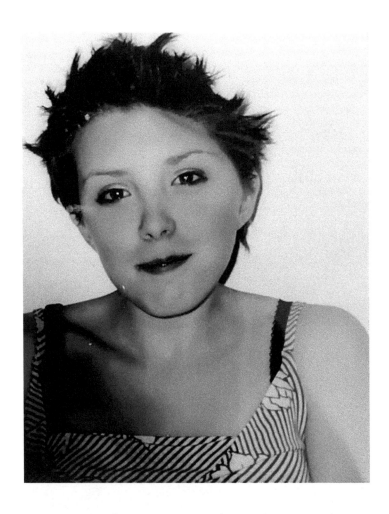

Waiting for my titanium plate to be inserted

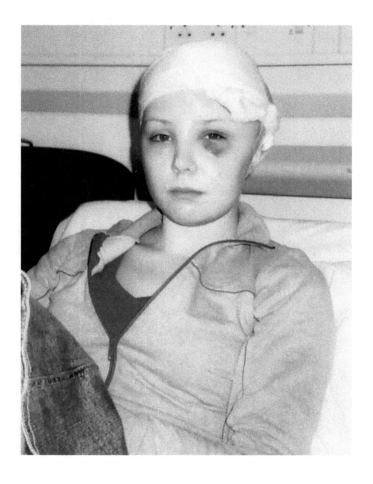

Finally, a whole head again!

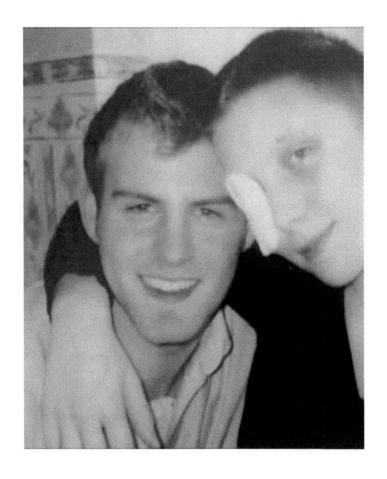

Andy and me, after my second operation

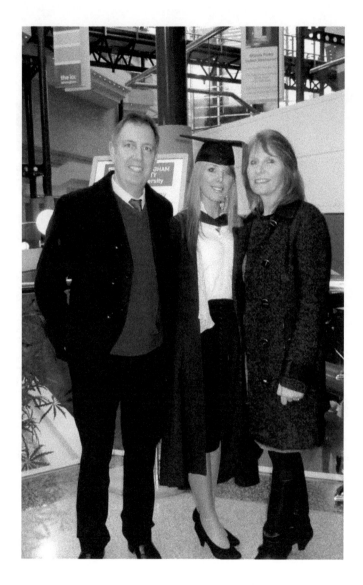

Graduation 2011 with Dad and Mum

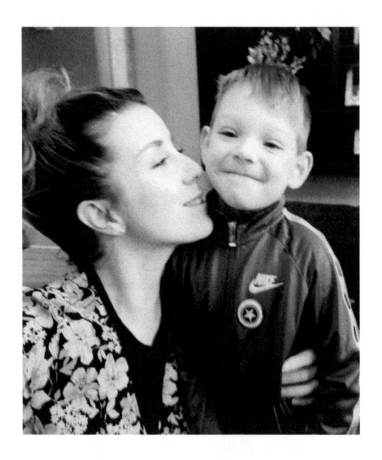

Me and my son. Happy days.

Resources

You can find out more about Gemma Bromley on her website and download some worksheets that have been discussed in this book:

www.gemmabromley.co.uk

You can also join Gemma's brain injury support group *Brain Dump!* on Facebook. This group is run in partnership with Rebekah Nesbitt. The group aims to support survivors and their family members to cope on a day to day basis, offering an optimistic look on life. As this group is new, we would love to hear from you, our mission is to reach out to as many people as we can – so please spread the love.

"When we support each other, and believe in our ideas - incredible things can happen" – Gemma Bromley

References

Chapter One: No Ordinary Morning
NHS Craniotomy: https://www.uhs.nhs.uk/OurServices/
Brainspineandneuromuscular/Neurosurgery/Diagnosi-
sandtreatment/Braintumours/Craniotomy.aspx

Chapter Two: Angel in a Coma
Barbato; 2002;Owen, A et al; 2006: https://oshosam-
masati.org/carers/rapport-skills/coma-communica-
tion-meditation/

NHS on Coma: https://www.nhs.uk/conditions/coma/

Chapter Three: Grey Matter
Know your brain: https://www.neuroscientificallychal-
lenged.com/blog/know-your-brain-wernickes-area

The role of Broca's area in speech perception:

https://www.ncbi.nlm.nih.gov/pmc/articles/
PMC3195945/

Brain injury on neglect: https://www.braininjury-explana-
tion.com/consequences/invisible-consequences/neglect

NHS Trust Dr. Paresh Malhotra: https://www.imperial.
nhs.uk/consultant-directory/paresh-malhotra

Chapter Four: Now Let Me Tell You

Headway UK: https://www.headway.org.uk/about-brain-injury/further-information/statistics/

Professor John Evans: Positive Psychology: https://www.cambridge.org/core/journals/brain-impairment/article/positive-psychology-and-brain-injury-rehabilitation/95AE2017B0076F291BA2E32DC5C430EE

Emilia Clarke: https://www.bbc.co.uk/news/av/entertainment-arts-48896472/emilia-clarke-backs-nhs-plan-to-support-young-stroke-survivors

Chapter Five: Baby Steps All the Way

Brainline: People with TBI: https://www.brainline.org/people-with-TBI

NHS: Brain Injury: https://www.nhs.uk/conditions/severe-head-injury/

Brainline: Flat affect: https://www.brainline.org/blog/learning-accident/impact-flat-affect-families-after-brain-injury

Chapter Six: The Tapestry of Life

Mirror Therapy: https://mirrortherapy.com/what-is-plasticity-of-the-brain-3/

NHS Morphine:

https://www.nhs.uk/medicines/morphine/

NHS Hallucinations: https://www.nhs.uk/conditions/hallucinations/

Chapter Seven: Everything Happens for a Reason

TRUTH Technique, Tina Gilbertston: https://tinagilbert-son.com/

Preventing Suicide in young people: https://papyrus-uk.org/

Ditch the label study: https://www.ditchthelabel.org/research-papers/the-annual-bullying-survey-2019/

Bullying in the workplace: https://www.bullying.co.uk/bullying-at-work/

Chapter Eight: What's Your Superpower?

Invisible disability: invisibledisabilitiesuk.weebly.com/

Different hidden disabilities: https://www.disabled-world.com/disability/types/invisible/

Famous people you'd never know had a disability: https://www.passionatepeople.invacare.eu.com/famous-disabled-people-inspire-day/

Still's disease: https://www.mayoclinic.org/diseases-conditions/adult-stills-disease/symptoms-causes/syc-20351907

Keira Knightly inspires people with dyslexia: https://www.dyslexia-reading-well.com/keira-knightley.html

Chapter Nine: Feel the Fear and Do It Anyway

NHS health and wellbeing: https://www.nwbh.nhs.uk/healthandwellbeing/Pages/Fight-or-Flight.aspx

Anxiety facts: https://www.mentalhealthy.co.uk/anxiety/anxiety/anxiety-facts-and-statistics.html

Chapter Ten: Not the F Word

Sleep and brain injury: https://msktc.org/tbi/factsheets/sleep-and-traumatic-brain-injury

Stages of sleep: https://www.webmd.com/sleep-disorders/sleep-101

Headway UK: wake up to fatigue: https://www.headway.org.uk/news-and-campaigns/campaigns/brain-drain-wake-up-to-fatigue/

Cognitive behavioural therapy after TBI: https://www.flintrehab.com/2019/cognitive-behavioral-therapy-after-traumatic-brain-injury/

Headway UK on diet: https://www.headway.org.uk/about-brain-injury/individuals/brain-injury-and-me/diet-after-brain-injury-healthy-body-healthy-mind/

Nutrition for Brain Injury: https://healthfully.com/435557-nutrition-for-a-brain-injury.html

Lightning Source UK Ltd.
Milton Keynes UK
UKHW021445030321
379714UK00011B/449